SHEET PAN
PALEO

200 ONE-TRAY RECIPES FOR QUICK PREPPING, EASY ROASTING AND HASSLE-FREE CLEAN UP

PAMELA ELLGEN

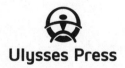

Ulysses Press

Published in the U.S. by
ULYSSES PRESS
P.O. Box 3440
Berkeley, CA 94703
www.ulyssespress.com

ISBN: 978-1-61243-523-7
Library of Congress Control Number: 2015944224

Printed in the United States by United Graphics, Inc.

10 9 8 7 6 5 4 3 2

Acquisitions Editor: Casie Vogel
Managing Editor: Claire Chun
Project Editor: Alice Riegert
Editor: Lauren Harrison
Proofreader: Barbara Schultz
Production: Caety Klingman
Front cover design: Michelle Thompson
Cover photographs: Pamela Ellgen

Distributed by Publishers Group West

NOTE TO READERS: This book has been written and published strictly for informational and educational purposes only. It is not intended to serve as medical advice or to be any form of medical treatment. You should always consult your physician before altering or changing any aspect of your medical treatment and/or undertaking a diet regimen, including the guidelines as described in this book. Do not stop or change any prescription medications without the guidance and advice of your physician. Any use of the information in this book is made on the reader's good judgment after consulting with his or her physician and is the reader's sole responsibility. This book is not intended to diagnose or treat any medical condition and is not a substitute for a physician.

This book is independently authored and published and no sponsorship or endorsement of this book by, and no affiliation with, any trademarked brands or other products mentioned within is claimed or suggested. All trademarks that appear in ingredient lists and elsewhere in this book belong to their respective owners and are used here for informational purposes only. The authors and publishers encourage readers to patronize the quality brands mentioned and pictured in this book.

To my mom, who was the first to say, "Don't toss the yolks!"
and raised me on a diet of whole foods. I am forever grateful for the
foundation of good nutrition she provided.

Contents

Introduction

When I first began eating Paleo foods, I thought the menu would be limited and that I would feel hungry all the time. Fortunately, my palate expanded to include a much wider variety of foods while my waistline shrunk, and best of all, I never felt hungry! Since then, I've explored the endless flavors available from meat, seafood, vegetables, fruit, nuts, and seeds, and discovered how delicious Paleo foods can be.

Sheet Pan Paleo offers a convenient solution to eating like your Paleolithic ancestors without spending hours hunting, fishing, or tending a fire—all with just a sheet pan! If you're like most of us, you stop by the market after a long workday, snag whatever's fresh, and head home to cook. This book makes it easy to prepare a filling Paleo meal.

The recipes are brimming with fresh vegetables, pastured meat and poultry, wild fish, and a generous dose of herbs and spices. There's even a bit of dark chocolate and wine thrown in for good measure. Recipes are naturally gluten- and dairy-free, and are labeled nightshade-free, vegan, and low-FODMAP, where applicable. FODMAPs are fermentable fibers found in a variety of foods that some people find difficult to digest.

Chapter 1 provides a general framework for Paleo foods. It contains guidance from experts on Paleo nutrition and evolutionary biology to help you understand the rationale behind the diet and how to choose the most nutritious foods within the Paleo paradigm.

The remaining chapters are arranged according to the main source of protein, from beef and lamb to fish and seafood, and there's even a chapter of all-vegetarian entrees. I've also included a chapter for appetizers and desserts. Recipes are easy to follow and designed to fit a whole meal onto one pan for easy preparation and cleanup. Some recipes are simple weeknight suppers to throw in the oven at a moment's notice, such as Plantain-Crusted Chicken Tenderloins with Steamed Carrots (page 93). Others are fit for a feast, such as Peppercorn-Crusted Beef Short Ribs with Sorrel and Radishes (page 148) or Roasted Chicken with Bacon-Glazed Brussels Sprouts and Caramelized Onions (page 96).

Whether you're new to Paleo cooking or a seasoned veteran, *Sheet Pan Paleo* appeals to your health goals and culinary sensibilities.

CHAPTER ONE
Paleo Basics

What Is Paleo?

Before the advent of agriculture, humans feasted on what they could hunt or gather—a diet of seasonal vegetables, fruit, and nuts, along with an array of eggs, game meats, wild fish, and even insects. The diet was complemented by regular physical activity and exposure to sunlight, the perils of prehistoric life notwithstanding.

Fast-forward to the modern landscape. Hunting and gathering is no longer a part of our lifestyle. Nevertheless, the unprocessed, whole plant and animal foods that humans consumed before the advent of agriculture, and specifically before the Industrial Revolution, are an ideal fuel. They provide the greatest nutrient density and the optimal ratios of macronutrients—fat, protein, and carbohydrate—for health and vitality.

Dr. Loren Cordain was one of the first to introduce a diet based on the Paleolithic period to a mainstream audience with his book *The Paleo Diet*. In an article published in the *American Journal of Clinical Nutrition*, he argued that Paleolithic diets varied widely based on geography, climate, and season, but necessarily would have included a diverse array of minimally processed, wild plant and animal foods and little or no grains, dairy, sugar, or industrial oils. Although there is some debate about exactly when humans began consuming these foods, it is clear that highly processed versions of these foods represent staples of modern life and that this is a drastic shift from the diets humans adapted to eating over many millennia. Numerous other researchers have contributed to the depth and breadth of knowledge on ancestral nutrition, including Robb Wolf, Mark Sisson, Chris Kresser, Paul Jaminet, PhD, Mat Lalonde PhD, and many other notable scientists. Their perspectives have been incorporated in choosing the ingredients and preparation methods in this book.

A Healthy Paradigm

I was first introduced to the Paleo diet by Aaron Blaisdell, PhD, professor at UCLA and founder of the Ancestral Health Symposium. One of the things I particularly appreciated about Dr. Blaisdell was his common-sense approach. He said, "The way to think about it is, 'What kinds of foods do humans thrive on, and which foods are dense with those kind of nutrients—the vitamins, minerals, and types of proteins—and in the optimal ratios? On the other end of the spectrum, which things are the most damaging?'"

Here is a general list of what not to eat on a Paleo-style diet:

- Processed foods
- Refined sugar
- High-fructose corn syrup
- Artificial sweeteners
- Industrial oils
- Legumes
- Grains
- Dairy

Here is a general list of foods you should eat on a Paleo-style diet:

- Vegetables and fruit
- Nuts and seeds
- Meat and poultry
- Organ meats
- Fish and shellfish
- Eggs
- Herbs and spices
- Vinegar and fermented foods

VEGETABLES AND FRUIT

Modern interpretations of the Paleo diet encourage choosing local, organic vegetables and fruit in season whenever possible. Frozen vegetables are a close second, but canned varieties are discouraged because they lose much of their nutritional value and are exposed to chemicals such as BPA from the can. I make an exception for canned tomatoes, but feel free to use fresh tomatoes if they're in season. Dried fruits are used with discretion because they're a concentrated source of sugar.

Here is a short list of vegetables and fruit available in each season, though the exact time frame varies based upon where you live:

Spring	Summer	Fall	Winter
Apricots	Apricots	Acorn squash	Beets
Artichokes	Beets	Asian pear	Belgian endive
Asparagus	Bell peppers	Belgian endive	Broccoli
Belgian endive	Blackberries	Broccoli	Brussels sprouts
Broccoli	Blueberries	Brussels sprouts	Cabbage
Butter lettuce	Butter lettuce	Butter Lettuce	Carrots
Cabbage	Cantaloupe	Butternut squash	Cauliflower
Chives	Corn	Cabbage	Celeriac
Collard greens	Cucumbers	Cauliflower	Clementines
Fennel	Eggplant	Cranberries	Collard greens
Green beans	Figs	Curly endive	Dates
Mango	Grapes	Garlic	Escarole
Mustard greens	Green beans	Ginger	Grapefruit
Onions	Jalapeños	Kumquats	Kale
Peas	Peaches	Kohlrabi	Kiwis
Radicchio	Peas	Mushrooms	Leeks
Red leaf lettuce	Radishes	Pears	Onions
Rhubarb	Raspberries	Persimmons	Oranges
Snow peas	Shallots	Plums	Parsnips
Sorrel	Sugar snap peas	Pumpkin	Pears
Spinach	Tomatillos	Radicchio	Pomegranates
Strawberries	Tomatoes	Sweet potatoes	Rutabagas
Swiss chard	Watermelon	Swiss chard	Sweet potatoes
Watercress	Zucchini	Turnips	Turnips

STARCHES

There is some debate within the Paleo community about starchy root vegetables such as sweet potatoes and white potatoes. The general consensus is that sweet potatoes deserve a place on your plate. White potatoes are often avoided because of toxins present in the skin and their high glycemic index. However, some Paleo proponents argue for white potatoes' inclusion, and I tend to agree, especially for people who need more carbohydrate than they typically get on a Paleo-style diet. Thus, a few recipes in this book include them. If you choose not to eat them, simply replace with sweet potatoes or choose an alternative recipe.

White rice is another gray area. It is a grain, and grains are universally avoided on the Paleo diet because they contain antinutrients and compounds that can irritate the lining of your gut. However, these substances are removed during the refining process, and you're left with pure starch. I have suggested white rice for serving with several dishes, but otherwise I haven't incorporated it into any recipes (e.g., as a filler for meatballs).

Ultimately, listen to your body and eat what makes you feel good, not to satisfy a specific approach to Paleo. See the resources section at the end of this book for more information on the Paleo approach.

NUTS AND SEEDS

Almonds, walnuts, pistachios, pecans, macadamia nuts, sesame seeds, sunflower seeds ... the list of nuts and seeds included on a Paleo diet is long. But it doesn't include peanuts, which are actually a legume. Choose raw nuts whenever possible to avoid those that have been roasted in inflammatory industrial oils. You may also wish to soak nuts overnight in fresh water and then rinse thoroughly to remove some enzymes that may cause digestive difficulties.

MEAT AND POULTRY

Choose organic, free-range, or pastured meat and poultry. Not only are the flavor and texture indescribably better, the meat is also far healthier for you, with a better composition of fatty acids and nutrients. Plus, the detrimental effects on the environment are minimized.

FISH AND SEAFOOD

Choose wild fish whenever possible. It has a better nutrient profile than farmed fish and is less devastating to ocean ecosystems. Consult the Monterey Bay Aquarium's Seafood Watch list to determine the best species and country of origin to purchase for the greatest nutrition and least environmental impact.

EGGS

The term "cage-free" on most supermarket eggs often means the chickens are crowded into an indoor barn with a small door to the outside world. If you can, purchase eggs from your local farmer's market, where you're more likely to find eggs from hens that actually had free range to eat bugs and bask in the sunshine.

FATS AND OILS

In this book, I call for olive oil in most recipes because that is what I use in cooking. Feel free to use a more heat-stable oil such as coconut or macadamia nut oil. You can also use butter (see "Dairy" on page 8). I also use rendered bacon fat in several recipes. I usually have some on hand, spooned from the breakfast pan and saved in the refrigerator until it is needed.

ORGAN MEATS

Organ meats such as heart, liver, and kidney are rich in vitamins and minerals. It is very important to choose offal (non-muscle meat) from pastured, sustainably raised and harvested animals. Organs tend to accumulate toxins, so conventionally farmed animal organs will be higher in these toxins.

VINEGAR AND FERMENTED FOODS

Fermented foods, such as sauerkraut, kimchi, and kombucha, possess myriad health benefits, including improved gut function and mental health. However, the beneficial effects are erased when fermented foods are heated above 115°F, thus no fermented foods are included in these recipes. If you wish to include them, use as condiments after cooking. I have included vinegar in many recipes, but primarily because it tastes good, not because of any specific health effect.

DAIRY

The jury is out on whether dairy is Paleo or not, but because I and so many other people just don't tolerate it well, I have not included it in this book. If you do enjoy dairy, choose organic, grass-fed, full-fat options, such as cream, butter or ghee, and full-fat yogurt and sour cream.

SUGAR

Paleo-friendly sweeteners include maple syrup, honey, and coconut palm sugar. I have used them in some sauces and in the dessert chapter. However, even these "healthy" sweeteners contain the same number of grams of sugar per teaspoon as does granulated sugar and should be enjoyed sparingly.

Cooking Equipment

For all of the recipes in this book, I used a 16½ x 12½ x 1-inch rimmed sheet pan. In restaurants, this is called a half sheet pan. A larger pan will work as well, but ensure that it has at least a 1-inch rim.

Many recipes call for lining the pan with parchment paper. This is typically for easy removal from the pan and to prevent food from burning on the metal. Whatever you do, don't use wax paper! It releases an unpleasant odor and sticks to many foods.

CHAPTER TWO

Appetizers & Sides

BROILED ROMAINE HEARTS WITH ROASTED RED PEPPERS AND OLIVES

My friend Julia introduced me to this amazing warm salad a few years ago, and it's been seared in my memory ever since. It's a delicious way to fill up on vegetables before your main course.

SERVES: 4   PREP TIME: 10 minutes   COOK TIME: 2 minutes

2 romaine lettuce hearts

2 tablespoons olive oil, divided

2 roasted red peppers, diced

¼ cup pitted kalamata olives

1 shallot or small red onion, thinly sliced

1 teaspoon fresh thyme leaves

juice of 1 lemon

sea salt

freshly ground pepper

1. Place the oven rack on the top level and preheat the broiler to high.

2. Slice the romaine hearts in half lengthwise and brush with 1 tablespoon of the olive oil. Set them on the sheet pan. Season with salt and pepper. Broil for 1 to 2 minutes, or until the top of the lettuce is lightly charred.

3. In a small bowl, combine the remaining olive oil, red peppers, olives, shallot, thyme, and lemon juice. Season with salt and pepper.

VEGAN

BALSAMIC RED CABBAGE

These tangy, savory, smoky cabbage slices will quickly become one of your favorite roasted vegetables. They are especially delicious with roasted chicken.

SERVES: 2 to 4   PREP TIME: 10 minutes   COOK TIME: 45 to 50 minutes

1 small red cabbage

¼ cup balsamic vinegar

2 teaspoons Dijon mustard

2 teaspoons ground cumin

2 tablespoons olive oil

sea salt

freshly ground pepper

1. Preheat the oven to 400°F. Line a sheet pan with parchment paper.

2. Slice the cabbage into 16 wedges, being sure to allow each one to retain a small portion of the core. This will help them hold together.

3. Whisk the balsamic, mustard, cumin, and oil together in a small bowl. Season with salt and pepper.

4. Lay the cabbage slices on the parchment paper. Drizzle with the balsamic vinaigrette.

5. Bake for 25 minutes before turning the cabbage over. Bake for another 20 to 25 minutes, until the cabbage is tender and gently browned.

NIGHTSHADE-FREE ▪ VEGAN

ROASTED GRAPE TOMATOES AND GARLIC

This can easily work as a deliciously savory side dish or be mashed gently with a fork and used to top your favorite Paleo pasta, such as zucchini noodles or almond flour pasta.

SERVES: 2 to 4   PREP TIME: 5 minutes   COOK TIME: 25 to 30 minutes

2 pints grape tomatoes

8 to 10 garlic cloves, smashed

2 tablespoons olive oil

1 teaspoon dried oregano

sea salt

freshly ground pepper

1. Preheat the oven to 375°F.

2. Spread the tomatoes and garlic out on a sheet pan. Drizzle with the olive oil and then season with the oregano, salt, and pepper.

3. Roast uncovered for 25 to 30 minutes, until the tomatoes are wilted and the garlic is golden.

VEGAN

SPICY MANGO CHUTNEY

This tangy condiment makes a perfect topping for vegetable chips or Sea Salt Almond Crackers (page 14). I also enjoy slathering it on meat during the last few minutes of cooking for a big boost of flavor.

SERVES: 4 to 6   PREP TIME: 10 minutes   COOK TIME: 30 to 45 minutes

1 red onion, diced

1 serrano chile, minced

1 red bell pepper, diced

2 mangoes, diced

2 tablespoons minced fresh ginger

¼ cup golden raisins

¼ cup apple cider vinegar

2 teaspoons curry powder

½ teaspoon ground cinnamon

½ teaspoon sea salt

2 tablespoons coconut palm sugar

1. Preheat the oven to 375°F. Line a sheet pan with parchment paper.

2. Place all of the ingredients in a medium bowl and toss to combine. Spread out on the sheet pan. Roast uncovered for 30 to 45 minutes, stirring occasionally, until the mango is soft and the onions are lightly caramelized.

VEGAN

SEA SALT ALMOND CRACKERS

Discovering the beauty of almond crackers was one of the best things that happened to me during my Paleo journey. They make the perfect snack to munch on while waiting for dinner and can be prepared and stored ahead of time. You're welcome to use almond meal instead of blanched almond flour. The texture will have a bit more grit, similar to whole wheat crackers.

MAKES: 24 crackers   PREP TIME: 5 minutes   COOK TIME: 15 minutes

2 cups blanched almond flour

½ teaspoon Himalayan pink sea salt, divided

1 tablespoon olive oil

2 to 3 tablespoons ice water

1. Preheat the oven to 325°F. Line a sheet pan with parchment paper.

2. Combine the almond flour and ¼ teaspoon of the sea salt in a food processor and pulse once or twice to combine.

3. Add the olive oil and 1 tablespoon of the ice water and pulse a few more times until a dough ball forms, adding additional water as necessary.

4. Place the dough on the sheet pan and cover with another sheet of parchment paper. Use a rolling pin to roll out the dough until it reaches the edges. The dough should be about ¹⁄₁₆-inch thick. Cut the crackers into 8 large pieces.

5. Bake uncovered for 10 minutes. Flip the pieces and move them around on the pan so that edge pieces are now near the center to allow for even browning. Sprinkle with the remaining sea salt and bake for another 5 minutes, or until the crackers are lightly browned.

NIGHTSHADE-FREE · LOW-FODMAP · VEGAN

CARAMELIZED ASPARAGUS

Asparagus becomes crunchy and sweet when roasted. Be careful, though—even a few minutes too long in the oven will give it a bitter char. For thick spears, increase the cooking time by 5 minutes.

SERVES: 2   PREP TIME: 5 minutes   COOK TIME: 20 to 25 minutes

1 bunch asparagus spears

2 tablespoons olive oil

1 tablespoon balsamic vinegar

sea salt

freshly ground pepper

1. Preheat the oven to 375°F. Line a sheet pan with parchment paper.

2. Spread the asparagus out on the sheet pan. Drizzle with the oil and vinegar and season with salt and pepper.

3. Cover the pan tightly with foil and bake for 15 minutes. Remove the foil for the last 5 to 10 minutes of cooking.

NIGHTSHADE-FREE ▪ LOW-FODMAP

RATATOUILLE

Thin slices of each vegetable allow the flavors to meld completely into a soft, succulent "pie filling" consistency. Serve as an appetizer with Sea Salt Almond Crackers (page 14) and an earthy red wine.

SERVES: 4   PREP TIME: 15 minutes   COOK TIME: 1½ hours

2 Japanese eggplants

2 plump zucchini

8 to 10 vine-ripened tomatoes

2 to 4 tablespoons olive oil, divided

2 tablespoons minced shallots

4 large garlic cloves, minced

1 cup fresh or canned tomato puree

2 sprigs fresh rosemary

4 sprigs fresh thyme

sea salt

freshly ground pepper

1. Slice the eggplant and zucchini in about ⅛-inch-thick slices. Sprinkle generously with salt, toss gently, and set aside in a colander to drain.

2. Slice the tomatoes in ⅛-inch slices as well.

3. Heat 2 tablespoons of olive oil over medium-low heat in a small skillet. Add the shallots and garlic with a pinch of salt, and cook, stirring, for about 4 minutes. Add the tomato puree and simmer on low heat for another few minutes.

4. Preheat the oven to 350°F.

5. Ladle the tomato sauce onto the sheet pan, adding oil as needed to coat the bottom of the dish.

6. Remove the eggplant and zucchini from the colander and pat dry with paper towels.

7. Layer the eggplant, zucchini, and tomato slices in the pan in a row pattern. Tuck in the sprigs of herbs among the vegetables and season with freshly ground pepper.

8. Cover tightly with foil and bake for about 1 hour. Remove the foil, drizzle with 2 tablespoons olive oil, and bake for another 30 to 45 minutes, until the vegetables begin to brown. Transfer to a cooling rack for about 15 minutes before plating.

9. To serve, create a stack of vegetables and top with a piece of thyme or rosemary. Spoon bits of the sauce around each plate.

VEGAN

SWEET POTATO OVEN FRIES

The secret to the best sweet potato fries lies in the technique—slice them thinly, toss in oil on the sheet pan, and then salt. Cook undisturbed until browned on the bottom and allow to cool for about 5 minutes before serving.

SERVES: 2 to 4   PREP TIME: 5 minutes   COOK TIME: 45 minutes

   4 to 6 small sweet potatoes, unpeeled

   2 to 4 tablespoons olive oil

   ¼ teaspoon sea salt

1. Preheat the oven to 375°F.

2. Use a mandoline or a sharp chef's knife to slice the sweet potatoes lengthwise into ½-inch thick slices, then slice into ½-inch-thick spears.

3. Place them on a rimmed sheet pan.

4. Drizzle with olive oil and toss to coat thoroughly.

5. Sprinkle with sea salt.

6. Bake for 45 minutes, or until the bottoms are brown and caramelized and the tops are soft and somewhat shriveled.

7. Season to taste with salt.

LOW-FODMAP · NIGHTSHADE-FREE

ROSEMARY PARSNIP FRIES

Parsnips and rosemary are a classic flavor combination, and for good reason! The evergreen aromas of rosemary beautifully offset the sweetness of the white root vegetable. Enjoy this quick and easy appetizer in the late fall when parsnips are at their peak.

SERVES: 2 to 4   PREP TIME: 5 minutes   COOK TIME: 20 minutes

4 parsnips, unpeeled

3 tablespoons olive oil

1 tablespoon minced fresh rosemary

sea salt

freshly ground pepper

1. Preheat the oven to 450°F.

2. Use a mandoline or a sharp chef's knife to slice the parsnips into ½-inch-thick spears.

3. Place them on a sheet pan.

4. Drizzle with olive oil and toss to coat thoroughly. Season generously with the rosemary, salt, and pepper.

5. Bake for 20 minutes, stirring halfway through.

LOW-FODMAP ▪ NIGHTSHADE-FREE

SWEET POTATO HOLIDAY DRESSING

This dish effectively re-creates the Thanksgiving favorite. It's grain- and gluten-free, and even suitable for the vegetarians at your table.

SERVES: 4   PREP TIME: 15 minutes   COOK TIME: 1 hour

2 large sweet potatoes, peeled

2 tablespoons minced fresh sage

2 tablespoons minced fresh parsley

1 tablespoon minced fresh thyme

4 tablespoons olive oil, divided

1 yellow onion, diced

3 celery stalks, diced

sea salt

freshly ground pepper

¼ cup vegetable broth

1. Preheat the oven to 375°F.

2. Cut the sweet potato into ½-inch dice. Toss with the herbs and 3 tablespoons of the oil and arrange on a sheet pan. Season generously with salt and pepper.

3. Roast uncovered for about 40 to 45 minutes, or until browned.

4. During the last 10 minutes of cooking, heat the remaining tablespoon of olive oil over medium-high heat in a large skillet and sauté the onion and celery until slightly softened.

5. When the sweet potatoes are finished baking, remove about 1 cup of them to a small bowl and mash gently with a potato masher or the back of a fork. This replicates the slightly smashed texture of traditional stuffing surprisingly well.

6. Add the mashed sweet potato back to the sheet pan, along with the sautéed onion and celery, tossing gently to combine.

7. Pour the broth over the dish, cover tightly with foil, and bake for another 15 minutes, or cool completely and bake until heated through when you're ready to serve.

NIGHTSHADE-FREE ▪ VEGAN

ROASTED CAULIFLOWER WITH PINE NUTS AND RAISINS

My husband, Rich, spent a week in Madrid on assignment and came back with stories of the many restaurants he visited. Naturally, this called for an evening of tapas. Because he doesn't eat meat, I explored some vegetarian options and stumbled upon this seriously awesome version of roasted cauliflower.

SERVES: 2 to 4   PREP TIME: 10 minutes   COOK TIME: 30 minutes

1 head cauliflower, broken or cut into small florets

2 garlic cloves, finely minced

zest and juice of 1 lemon

¼ cup olive oil

¼ cup pine nuts

½ cup raisins

¼ cup roughly chopped fresh parsley

sea salt

freshly ground pepper

1. Preheat the oven to 375°F.

2. In a large mixing bowl, combine the cauliflower with the garlic, lemon zest, and olive oil. Spread out over the sheet pan. Season generously with salt and pepper. Roast for 30 minutes uncovered, or until the cauliflower browns on the bottom and shrivels slightly.

3. Meanwhile, toast the pine nuts in a dry skillet over medium-low heat for 2 to 4 minutes, or until fragrant and golden brown.

4. Toss the roasted cauliflower together with the pine nuts and raisins and then shower with parsley and lemon juice. Serve warm.

NIGHTSHADE-FREE

PROSCIUTTO-WRAPPED DATES

These are my absolute favorite tapas, and they're a cinch to make. Dates are packed with sugar, so they're awesome after an endurance workout or when you just want to splurge.

SERVES: 4 to 6   PREP TIME: 10 minutes   COOK TIME: 15 to 20 minutes

- 16 medjool dates, pitted
- 16 Marcona almonds
- 8 slices prosciutto, halved lengthwise

1. Preheat the oven to 350°F. Line a sheet pan with parchment paper.

2. Tuck a single almond into each of the dates. Wrap the date with the prosciutto and place with the "seam" side down on the sheet pan.

3. Bake for 15 to 20 minutes, or until the prosciutto is barely crispy.

NIGHTSHADE-FREE • LOW-FODMAP

STUFFED PEARS WITH PROSCIUTTO

I enjoyed this recipe originally with Gorgonzola and cream cheese and loved it. Unfortunately, dairy doesn't love me back, so I had to come up with a dairy-free version. This one may just be better than the original. It's a delicious appetizer or delightful as a side dish for brunch.

SERVES: 4   PREP TIME: 10 minutes   COOK TIME: 15 minutes

4 ripe pears, halved lengthwise and cored

½ cup toasted macadamia nuts

2 pitted medjool dates

1 teaspoon minced fresh rosemary

¼ teaspoon sea salt

1 tablespoon port or sweet red wine

4 slices prosciutto, halved crosswise

1. Preheat the oven to 400°F. Line a sheet pan with parchment paper.

2. Spread the pears cut-side up on the sheet pan. You may have to cut a small portion off the bottom of each one so they don't tip over.

3. Pulse the macadamia nuts in a food processor until coarsely ground. Add the dates, rosemary, sea salt, and port. Pulse until thoroughly combined.

4. Divide the mixture among the pears and top each with a slice of prosciutto. Bake for 15 minutes, or until the prosciutto is crisp and the pears gently softened.

NIGHTSHADE-FREE

ROASTED EGGPLANT

This recipe looks like it contains a lot of olive oil, but trust me, it's worth it. It helps the interior of the eggplant break down into a succulent, creamy consistency and the outside to get brown and crispy.

SERVES: 2 to 4   PREP TIME: 10 minutes   COOK TIME: 40 to 45 minutes

½ cup olive oil

zest of 1 lemon

2 garlic cloves, minced

¼ cup minced fresh parsley

2 medium eggplants, sliced in ¼-inch-thick slices

sea salt

freshly ground pepper

2 tablespoons red wine vinegar

1. Preheat the oven to 375°F.

2. Combine the olive oil, lemon zest, garlic, and parsley in a small mixing bowl. Dredge each of the eggplant slices in the mixture and set on a sheet pan. Season generously with salt and pepper.

3. Roast uncovered for 40 to 45 minutes or until the center of the eggplant is thoroughly wilted and the bottoms of each slice is browned.

4. Serve warm and sprinkle with red wine vinegar just before serving.

VEGAN

CARAMELIZED FENNEL

Oven roasting has a way of transforming vegetables into something entirely different from their raw states, and it is especially true with fennel bulb. Raw, fennel is crunchy and peppery, with a prominent licorice or anise flavor. Roasted, it becomes creamy with a subtle, mellow flavor.

SERVES: 4 to 6   PREP TIME: 5 minutes   COOK TIME: 40 to 45 minutes

2 fennel bulbs

¼ cup olive oil

sea salt

freshly ground pepper

1 tablespoon sherry vinegar, for serving

1. Preheat the oven to 375°F.

2. Cut the bottom off of each fennel bulb then cut into quarters. Remove any tough exterior pieces and the core. Reserve the fennel fronds. Slice each quarter into two slices, yielding eight pieces per bulb. Place the slices on a sheet pan. Toss with olive oil and season generously with salt and pepper.

3. Roast for 45 to 50 minutes, or until browned around the edges. To serve, douse with sherry vinegar and top with the fennel fronds.

NIGHTSHADE-FREE ▪ VEGAN

ROASTED BEETS WITH MUSTARD AND TARRAGON

Beets pair beautifully with mustard and tarragon in this simple side dish.

SERVES: 4   PREP TIME: 5 minutes   COOK TIME: 40 minutes

4 to 6 small to medium beets, peeled

2 tablespoons olive oil

pinch of sea salt

2 tablespoons honey

2 tablespoons champagne vinegar

½ teaspoon Dijon mustard

1 tablespoon minced fresh tarragon

1. Preheat the oven to 350°F.

2. Cut the beets into quarters and toss with the olive oil and sea salt on a sheet pan.

3. Roast uncovered for 40 minutes.

4. In a small bowl, whisk together the honey, vinegar, mustard, and tarragon.

5. When the beets have finished cooking, toss them with the dressing. Allow the flavors to come together for 5 to 10 minutes. Serve warm or chilled.

NIGHTSHADE-FREE ▪ VEGAN

SAUSAGE-STUFFED MUSHROOM CAPS

Typical stuffed mushrooms rely on bread crumbs to soak up excess moisture. This Paleo-friendly version uses low-moisture, filling ingredients and some coconut flour to do the job.

SERVES: 4 to 6   PREP TIME: 15 minutes   COOK TIME: 15 minutes

1 teaspoon olive oil

1 cup finely diced yellow onion

½ pound Italian sausage, casings removed

1 roasted red pepper, minced

1 tablespoon minced parsley

2 teaspoons coconut flour

sea salt

1 egg, whisked

3 dozen cremini mushrooms

1. Preheat the oven to 375°F. Line a sheet pan with parchment paper.

2. Warm the oil in a large skillet over medium heat. Add the onion and a pinch of sea salt, allowing the onions to release their moisture and cook down for 10 minutes. Push the onions to the side of the pan, add the sausage, and brown for about 2 minutes.

3. Transfer the onion and sausage mixture to a large bowl and add the red pepper, parsley, and coconut flour. Season with salt. Add the egg and incorporate all of the filling ingredients with your hands.

4. Remove the stems from the mushrooms and reserve for another use. Clean the mushrooms of dirt and debris. Place them gill-side up on the sheet pan and fill each with about 1 tablespoon of the filling.

5. Bake uncovered for 20 minutes, or until the tops are browned and the mushrooms wilted.

TURNIPS AND PEARS WITH THYME

This side dish is comfort food at its finest. Enjoy as an appetizer or with a whole roasted chicken, which you can cut butterfly, or "spatchcock," and cook right on top.

SERVES: 4   PREP TIME: 10 minutes   COOK TIME: 35 to 40 minutes

4 turnips, peeled and chopped in 1- to 2-inch pieces

2 pears, cored and cut into 1- to 2-inch pieces

2 tablespoons olive oil

1 sprig thyme, leaves only

sea salt

freshly ground pepper

1. Preheat the oven to 375°F. Line a sheet pan with parchment paper.

2. Spread the turnips and pears out on the sheet pan and toss gently with the olive oil. Sprinkle with the thyme and season generously with salt and pepper.

3. Roast uncovered for 35 to 40 minutes, or until the turnips are browned and soft.

NIGHTSHADE-FREE · VEGAN

ACORN SQUASH WITH SAGE AND HAZELNUTS

I grew up enjoying roasted acorn squash topped with butter and brown sugar for breakfast. This savory version is just as delicious.

SERVES: 4   PREP TIME: 5 minutes   COOK TIME: 45 minutes

2 acorn squash, halved lengthwise

2 tablespoons coconut palm sugar

1 sprig fresh sage

¼ teaspoon sea salt

1 tablespoon coconut oil, melted

¼ cup toasted hazelnuts, roughly chopped

1. Preheat the oven to 375°F. Line a sheet pan with parchment paper.

2. Place the acorn squash cut-side down on the sheet pan. Roast for 30 minutes.

3. Meanwhile, combine the palm sugar, sage, and sea salt in a mortar and pestle until thoroughly combined.

4. Remove the squash from the oven and turn them over. Brush each with coconut oil and then sprinkle with the sage and coconut sugar mixture. Return to the oven to roast, uncovered, for another 10 to 15 minutes, or until lightly browned and bubbling. Top with the crushed hazelnuts to serve.

NIGHTSHADE-FREE ▪ **VEGAN**

FIERY BARBECUE CHICKEN WINGS

Nothing says party food quite like barbecue chicken wings. But the atmosphere is far less festive if you read the ingredients in most commercially prepared barbecue sauces: soybean oil, sodium benzoate, and natural butter-type flavor. No thanks!

SERVES: 4 to 6   PREP TIME: 10 minutes   COOK TIME: 40 minutes

½ cup coconut oil

¼ cup red wine vinegar

1 tablespoon ancho chile powder

1 teaspoon cayenne pepper

1 teaspoon smoked paprika

2 garlic cloves

1 tablespoon maple syrup

2 pounds chicken wings

sea salt

4 to 6 celery stalks, for serving

1. Preheat the oven to 375°F. Line a sheet pan with parchment paper.

2. To make the barbecue sauce, combine the oil, vinegar, spices, garlic, and maple syrup in a blender and puree until smooth. Season to taste with salt.

3. Place the sauce and chicken wings in a large bowl, tossing to coat. Spread out on the sheet pan and roast uncovered for 40 minutes, or until cooked through.

4. Allow to cool for at least 10 minutes, then serve with the celery stalks.

PESTO ROASTED ZUCCHINI

Summertime flavors combine for a light and healthy appetizer.

SERVES: 4 to 6   PREP TIME: 15 minutes   COOK TIME: 25 to 30 minutes

6 zucchini

¼ cup olive oil

¼ cup pine nuts, toasted

1 cup fresh basil

2 garlic cloves

sea salt

freshly ground pepper

1. Preheat the oven to 425°F. Line a sheet pan with parchment paper.

2. Halve the zucchini lengthwise and scoop out the seeds with a spoon or melon baller.

3. Combine the olive oil, pine nuts, basil, and garlic in a blender and pulse until combined but still somewhat chunky. Season to taste with salt and pepper.

4. Divide the pesto mixture between the zucchini and bake uncovered for 25 to 30 minutes. Allow to cool for at least 10 minutes before serving.

NIGHTSHADE-FREE ▪ VEGAN

BEET AND PARSNIP CHIPS

There's something sublime about biting into a crunchy chip dipped into a bowl of cold ceviche or roasted red pepper dip. Unfortunately, most of the commercially prepared root vegetable chips use canola oil, an industrial oil not included on the Paleo menu. Try these chips instead.

SERVES: 2 to 4   PREP TIME: 15 minutes   COOK TIME: 15 minutes

2 parsnips, unpeeled	sea salt
2 beets, peeled	2 tablespoons coconut oil

1. Preheat the oven to 375°F. Line a sheet pan with parchment paper.

2. Slice the parsnips and beets into 1/16-inch-thick slices with a mandoline or a sharp chef's knife. Toss them with a generous pinch of sea salt and allow to rest in a colander for about 10 to 15 minutes. Blot them dry with a paper towel, then toss them into a large bowl with the coconut oil, ensuring all slices are coated.

3. Spread the vegetable slices on the sheet pan and roast uncovered for about 15 minutes, or until just crisp and beginning to brown. Be careful not to overbake. You will have to do this in batches. Allow to cool on a cooling rack, and then store in an airtight container for up to three days.

NIGHTSHADE-FREE ▪ VEGAN

BROILED OYSTERS WITH BACON, MUSHROOMS, AND SHALLOTS

Nothing says "Paleo" quite like bacon and oysters. This dish is so nutrient-dense, you might just want to enjoy these for dinner with a side of mixed greens. Although they do require a bit of advance preparation, the actual cooking time is minimal and the flavors are awesome!

SERVES: 4   PREP TIME: 20 minutes   COOK TIME: 2 minutes

4 slices applewood-smoked bacon, cut into small pieces

½ cup minced fresh button mushrooms

1 teaspoon fresh thyme

1 shallot, minced

1 teaspoon sherry vinegar

1 dozen oysters

1. Cook the bacon in a medium skillet over medium-low heat until most of the fat is rendered. Add the mushrooms, thyme, and shallot and cook for another 5 minutes, or until the mushrooms have released their moisture and some of it has evaporated. Splash with the sherry vinegar.

2. Scrub and rinse the oysters thoroughly using a vegetable brush. One at a time, place them in a dish towel and use an oyster knife to pry the shells apart. Be careful not to damage the meat or pour the juice out. Slide the knife beneath the meat to dislodge it from the shell. Repeat with the remaining oysters.

3. Place an oven rack on the top shelf and preheat the broiler to high.

4. Arrange the oysters on the sheet pan, and use crumpled aluminum foil to support them so they do not tip over. Top each oyster with a spoonful of the bacon and mushroom mixture.

5. Broil for 2 minutes, until the bacon mixture is browned and bubbling.

NIGHTSHADE-FREE

COCONUT SHRIMP WITH SPICY CHILI DIPPING SAUCE

Is there any dish more ubiquitous to the chain restaurant appetizer menu than coconut shrimp? Unfortunately, it's usually dredged in flour, fried in denatured industrial oil, and then served with a sticky sweet sauce. Whether you follow a Paleo diet or not, my take on the classic app is far healthier.

SERVES: 4   PREP TIME: 10 minutes   COOK TIME: 10 to 12 minutes

1 pound large shrimp, butterflied

2 egg whites

½ teaspoon sea salt

½ teaspoon garlic powder

½ teaspoon smoked paprika

1 cup unsweetened shredded coconut

1 tablespoon hot sauce

¼ cup maple syrup

1 tablespoon apple cider vinegar

1. Preheat the oven to 425°F. Line a sheet pan with parchment paper.

2. Whisk the egg whites with the salt, garlic powder, and paprika until frothy. Dip each of the shrimp into the egg white mixture, allowing any excess to drip back into the bowl. Press each shrimp into the shredded coconut, making sure it is coated on all sides. Place on the sheet pan and repeat with the remaining shrimp.

3. Bake for 10 to 12 minutes, or until the shrimp are cooked through and the coconut is lightly browned.

4. Meanwhile, whisk together the hot sauce, maple syrup, and vinegar. Serve alongside the shrimp.

SPICED MIXED NUTS

You really don't know the beauty of spiced nuts until you've made your own. If you're like me, you probably burned your fingers, as you couldn't resist trying them straight from the pan! If you soak your nuts before cooking, allow them to air-dry on a rack before mixing with the spices.

MAKES: 4 cups   PREP TIME: 5 minutes   COOK TIME: 10 to 15 minutes

1 cup pecans

1 cup cashews

1 cup almonds

1 cup Brazil nuts

⅓ cup coconut oil

¼ cup coconut palm sugar

2 tablespoons hot sauce, such as Cholula

1 teaspoon sea salt

1. Preheat the oven to 350°F. Line a sheet pan with parchment paper.

2. Combine the nuts in a large bowl. In a separate small bowl, whisk together the oil, palm sugar, hot sauce, and sea salt. Pour over the nuts and toss to coat thoroughly.

3. Spread the mixture out over the sheet pan and bake for 10 to 15 minutes, stirring once. Allow to cool thoroughly before enjoying.

LOW-FODMAP ▪ VEGAN

CHAPTER 3

Vegetarian

ROASTED SWEET POTATO BISQUE

You can easily make your own broth for this hearty soup by simmering vegetable scraps in water for an hour or two with a generous pinch of sea salt. For a flavorful broth, I use mushrooms, fennel, bell pepper, carrots, onions, celery, and tomato. Typically, I'll save these scraps over the course of a few weeks in a bag in the freezer until I need broth for a recipe. It's frugal and sustainable—a win-win if you ask me.

SERVES: 2 to 4   PREP TIME: 10 minutes   COOK TIME: 30 minutes

2 large sweet potatoes, peeled

1 yellow onion

1 Granny Smith apple

2 tablespoons coconut oil

sea salt

1 tablespoon curry powder

¼ cup coconut cream

4 cups (32 ounces) vegetable broth, heated

fresh cilantro, for serving

1. Preheat the oven to 375°F. Line a sheet pan with parchment paper.

2. Peel the sweet potatoes and cut into 1-inch chunks. Peel the onion and cut into large chunks. Peel and core the apple and cut into wedges. Place the vegetables on the sheet pan and drizzle with coconut oil. Season with salt.

3. Roast uncovered for 30 minutes, or until fork tender but not overly browned.

4. Place the cooked vegetables in a blender and add the curry powder, coconut cream, and just enough vegetable broth to loosen things up. Blend until smooth. Add the remaining broth and pulse until just combined. You may have to do this in two batches depending upon the size of your blender.

5. Serve with fresh cilantro.

VEGAN

ROASTED PARSNIP SOUP WITH POMEGRANATE

Choose parsnips in late fall after the first frost when the starches have naturally converted to sugars to yield a sweet root vegetable.

SERVES: 2 to 4   PREP TIME: 10 minutes   COOK TIME: 30 minutes

6 parsnips, unpeeled

2 shallots

2 tablespoons coconut oil, melted

1 tablespoon minced fresh rosemary

¼ cup coconut cream

4 cups (32 ounces) vegetable broth, heated

arils of 1 pomegranate

sea salt

1. Preheat the oven to 375°F. Line a sheet pan with parchment paper.

2. Cut the parsnips into 1-inch chunks. Peel the shallots and slice into quarters. Place the vegetables on the sheet pan and drizzle with coconut oil. Season with salt.

3. Roast for 30 minutes, or until fork tender but not overly browned.

4. Place the cooked vegetables in a blender and add the rosemary, coconut cream, and just enough vegetable broth to loosen things up. Blend until smooth. Add the remaining broth and pulse until just combined.

5. To serve, sprinkle the pomegranate arils over each portion of soup.

NIGHTSHADE-FREE ▪ VEGAN

ROASTED CAULIFLOWER BISQUE

Cauliflower florets become crunchy, sweet, and delicious when roasted. This soup uses these pieces as a topping for the soup, providing textural contrast.

SERVES: 2 to 4   PREP TIME: 10 minutes   COOK TIME: 45 minutes

1 head cauliflower

¼ cup coconut oil or ghee

2 garlic cloves, minced

zest and juice of 1 lemon

1 (15-ounce) can coconut milk

4 cups (32 ounces) vegetable broth, heated

¼ cup roughly chopped fresh parsley

sea salt

freshly ground pepper

1. Preheat the oven to 400°F.

2. Break the cauliflower into florets and place into a large bowl with the oil, garlic, and lemon zest. Toss to combine. Season generously with salt and pepper. Spread out on a sheet pan.

3. Roast uncovered for 35 to 45 minutes, or until the cauliflower is fork tender.

4. Divide the cauliflower, placing the tender but not browned pieces into a blender. Reserve the smaller browned pieces for garnish. If none are browned, return the pan to the oven to cook those small pieces for another 5 to 10 minutes.

5. Place the cooked cauliflower in a blender and add the coconut milk, vegetable broth, and lemon juice. Blend until smooth. Season to taste with salt and pepper.

6. To serve, garnish each serving with fresh parsley and the browned cauliflower bits.

NIGHTSHADE-FREE • VEGAN

ROASTED VEGETABLE FRITTATA

This is one of my favorite recipes to make on the last day before grocery shopping. Nearly any root vegetable or herb combination will work, so whatever needs to be cleaned out of your pantry or vegetable drawer is a good candidate.

SERVES: 4   PREP TIME: 10 minutes   COOK TIME: 50 minutes

6 to 8 cups assorted vegetables, such as sweet potatoes, beets, carrots, fennel, parsnips, and onions

2 tablespoons minced fresh parsley

2 teaspoons minced fresh rosemary

¼ cup olive oil

1 dozen eggs

sea salt

freshly ground black pepper

1. Preheat the oven to 375°F.

2. Cut the vegetables into 1- to 2-inch pieces. Toss them with the herbs and olive oil on a rimmed sheet pan. Season with salt and pepper. Roast uncovered for 40 minutes, or until soft and caramelized around the edges.

3. Combine the eggs in a large pitcher or bowl and whisk until nearly combined. Season with salt.

4. Pour the eggs into the sheet pan and return to the oven for 10 to 12 minutes, or until the eggs are nearly set. Allow to rest for 5 minutes before cutting and serving.

NIGHTSHADE-FREE

SUNDRIED TOMATO AND MUSHROOM FRITTATA

The flavors of roasted mushrooms and sundried tomatoes add complexity to this frittata. It's delicious for dinner, but would also make a fantastic brunch dish.

SERVES: 4   PREP TIME: 10 minutes   COOK TIME: 40 minutes

4 cups cremini mushrooms (about 16 ounces)

1 tablespoon olive oil

1 cup sundried tomatoes in olive oil, roughly chopped

2 tablespoons minced fresh parsley

2 green onions, sliced thinly on a bias

1 dozen eggs

sea salt

freshly ground pepper

1. Preheat the oven to 375°F.

2. Cut the mushrooms into quarters and toss with the olive oil on a rimmed sheet pan. Sprinkle with the sundried tomatoes, parsley, and green onions. Season with salt and pepper. Roast uncovered for 20 minutes.

3. Combine the eggs in a large pitcher or bowl and whisk until nearly combined. Season with salt.

4. Pour the eggs into the sheet pan and return to the oven for 10 to 12 minutes, or until the eggs are nearly set. Allow to rest for 5 minutes before cutting and serving.

NIGHTSHADE-FREE

SPAGHETTI SQUASH WITH ROASTED VEGETABLES

I think I was the very last person to discover how awesome spaghetti squash is. I cooked it for the first time, raked a fork through it, and gasped—it actually looked like spaghetti! Go figure. This version is completely vegan and oh so satisfying.

SERVES: 4   PREP TIME: 10 minutes   COOK TIME: 30 to 35 minutes

2 spaghetti squashes, about 1½ pounds each, cut in half lengthwise

¼ cup olive oil, divided

1 pint grape tomatoes

1 head garlic, cloves peeled

2 zucchini, halved then cut into 1-inch pieces

1 cup roughly chopped fresh basil

sea salt

freshly ground pepper

1. Preheat the oven to 375°F.

2. Remove the seeds from the spaghetti squash. Rub with a few teaspoons of olive oil and season with salt. Place cut-side down on the sheet pan.

3. Toss the tomatoes, garlic, and zucchini with the remaining oil and scatter it around the spaghetti squash on the pan. Season generously with salt and pepper.

4. Roast uncovered for 30 to 35 minutes. Place the spaghetti squash halves on individual plates and scrape with a fork to create long strands.

5. Toss the remaining vegetables with the fresh basil and divide between the squashes.

VEGAN

CAULIFLOWER PIZZA WITH PEPPERS, OLIVES, AND ARTICHOKE HEARTS

Most cauliflower pizza crusts rely on Parmesan cheese as a binder, but many people cannot eat dairy, so this version uses on egg, flax meal, and almond flour to hold it together. Top the pizza with whatever you like, or go with my favorites: roasted red peppers, artichoke hearts, and kalamata olives.

SERVES: 2 to 4   PREP TIME: 15 minutes   COOK TIME: 20 to 25 minutes

1 large head cauliflower

3 garlic cloves, minced

1 tablespoon olive oil

1 tablespoon Italian herb blend

1 egg

1 tablespoon flax meal

1 tablespoon blanched almond flour

½ teaspoon sea salt

1 cup prepared marinara sauce

2 roasted red bell peppers, sliced thinly

½ cup pitted kalamata olives, roughly chopped

1 cup artichoke hearts, quartered

½ red onion, sliced in thin rings

freshly ground pepper

1. Preheat the oven to 400°F. Cut a sheet of parchment paper to fit the sheet pan and go up the sides.

2. Cut the cauliflower using your food processor with the grater attachment. Place all of the grated cauliflower in a large baking dish and microwave for 4 minutes, stirring halfway through. Allow the cooked cauliflower to rest for about 5 minutes, stirring occasionally, until it is cool enough to handle.

3. Meanwhile, whisk together the garlic, olive oil, herb blend, egg, flax meal, almond flour, and sea salt. Season with pepper.

4. Squeeze all of the moisture out of the cauliflower. I find that a nut milk bag is the easiest, cleanest method, but if you do not have one, you can also use a clean dish towel to wring all of the moisture out of it.

5. Stir the cauliflower into the egg mixture until thoroughly combined. Press it into the sheet pan, covering the bottom and going up the sides slightly.

6. Bake uncovered for 15 minutes, or until golden brown.

7. Top with marinara sauce then peppers, olives, artichoke hearts, and onions, and bake for another 5 to 10 minutes.

SAGE AND GARLIC STUFFED SWEET POTATOES

Fall is my favorite season for comfort foods, and these twice-baked sweet potatoes fit the bill. They have all of the delicious flavors of the season. I recommend planning two sweet potatoes per person unless you're going to serve a salad or a side dish.

SERVES: 4   PREP TIME: 15 minutes   COOK TIME: 1 hour and 15 minutes

8 small sweet potatoes

1 head garlic

2 tablespoons plus 1 teaspoon coconut oil, divided

½ cup hazelnuts

2 tablespoons minced fresh sage, divided

sea salt

freshly ground pepper

1. Preheat the oven to 350°F.

2. Poke each of the sweet potatoes several times with the tines of a fork. Place them on the sheet pan.

3. Cut the top off of the head of garlic, place on a square of aluminum foil, drizzle with a teaspoon of coconut oil, and wrap into a small package. Place on the sheet pan.

4. Roast the sweet potatoes and garlic for 45 minutes. Remove from the oven. Slice the sweet potatoes nearly in half lengthwise, leaving the skins intact. Open the package of garlic and allow it all to rest for 15 minutes.

5. Meanwhile, roast the hazelnuts on the sheet pan for 10 to 15 minutes, being careful not to overcook. Remove from the oven and wrap in a dish towel. Allow to rest briefly and then rub the nuts between the layers of the towel to remove the skins.

6. When the sweet potatoes and garlic are cool enough to handle, scoop the flesh of the sweet potatoes into a large bowl. Squeeze each of the garlic cloves into the bowl and add the coconut oil and 1½ tablespoons of the sage. Stir gently to combine and season with salt and pepper. Divide the mixture among the sweet potato skins. Top with the remaining sage. Bake for another 15 minutes.

7. Roughly chop the hazelnuts and sprinkle them over the sweet potatoes just before serving.

NIGHTSHADE-FREE ▪ VEGAN

MAPLE ROASTED BEET SALAD WITH PEPITAS

Play up the natural sweetness of beets with a touch of maple syrup balanced with red wine vinegar for a simple appetizer or side dish. Make a chiffonade of the beet greens to add to the mixed greens. They're full of micronutrients and it's a great way to use up the whole vegetable.

SERVES: 4   PREP TIME: 5 minutes   COOK TIME: 40 minutes

½ cup pepitas (pumpkin seeds),

4 to 6 small to medium beets, peeled

2 tablespoons olive oil

pinch of sea salt

¼ cup maple syrup

¼ cup red wine vinegar

8 cups mixed greens

freshly ground pepper

1. Preheat the oven to 350°F.

2. In a small skillet, toast the pepitas over medium-high heat for about 5 minutes until fragrant. Set aside to cool.

3. Cut the beets into quarters and toss with the olive oil and a pinch of sea salt on the sheet pan.

4. Roast uncovered for 30 minutes. Drizzle with the maple syrup and vinegar, tossing gently to coat. Return to the oven to cook for another 10 minutes.

5. Allow the cooked beets to rest for 10 minutes, then divide them among four plates of mixed greens. Spoon the remaining pan juices over the salads and then top with toasted pepitas. Season with sea salt and freshly ground pepper.

NIGHTSHADE-FREE ▪ LOW-FODMAP ▪ VEGAN

BAKED EGGS IN AVOCADO WITH SMOKY SWEET POTATOES

This makes a delightful Paleo breakfast or dinner, and the eggs and avocado look so pretty together! You could certainly serve this without the sweet potatoes, but they keep the avocados from tipping over in the oven.

SERVES: 2 to 4   PREP TIME: 5 minutes   COOK TIME: 25 to 30 minutes

2 medium sweet potatoes, peeled, diced

2 tablespoons olive oil

2 garlic cloves, minced

1 teaspoon smoked paprika

2 avocados

4 medium eggs

sea salt

freshly ground pepper

1. Preheat the oven to 425°F.

2. Combine the diced sweet potatoes with the olive oil, garlic, and smoked paprika. Season generously with salt and pepper. Spread them evenly over the sheet pan and roast uncovered for 10 minutes.

3. Meanwhile, slice the avocados lengthwise and remove the pits. If the cavity looks too small to hold the egg, scoop out some of the avocado flesh and reserve it for another use.

4. Remove the sweet potatoes from the oven. Carefully place the avocado halves on the sweet potatoes, cut-side up. Crack an egg into each one. Season with salt and pepper. Return to the oven for 15 to 20 minutes, or until the egg white is set. Allow to rest for 5 minutes before serving.

SWEET POTATO HASH WITH BAKED EGGS

This recipe is also a winner for breakfast or for dinner. I typically purchase bags of small sweet potatoes, about 4 inches long. If you're using larger root vegetables, two may be enough.

SERVES: 2 to 4   PREP TIME: 15 minutes   COOK TIME: 45 minutes

3 sweet potatoes, peeled, diced

1 yellow onion, halved then sliced in thin half circles

1 green bell pepper, sliced in long strips

2 roasted red peppers, diced

2 tablespoons fresh parsley

2 tablespoons olive oil

4 to 6 eggs

1. Preheat the oven to 375°F.

2. Combine all of the ingredients except the eggs on the sheet pan. Season generously with salt and pepper, tossing gently to combine. Roast uncovered for 20 minutes.

3. Remove the pan from the oven. Make a small well in the roasted vegetables for each egg. Crack the eggs into each space and return to the oven for 15 minutes, or until the egg whites are set. Use a metal spatula to carefully remove each egg and the vegetables that surround it to individual serving plates.

ZUCCHINI AND SWEET POTATO FRITTERS WITH CHIPOTLE AIOLI

This works equally well as an appetizer and is a way to sneak veggies into an otherwise meat-heavy meal. Although these fritters won't hold up quite like dense fritters glued together with wheat flour, they're loaded with flavor and are best enjoyed with a fork and knife.

SERVES: 2   PREP TIME: 10 minutes   COOK TIME: 30 minutes

2 cups shredded unpeeled sweet potato

2 cups shredded zucchini

2 garlic cloves, minced

1 small onion, sliced in thin half circles

1 egg, whisked

¼ cup Paleo Mayonnaise (page 251)

juice of 1 lime

1 tablespoon minced chipotle in adobo

¼ cup roughly chopped fresh cilantro

sea salt

freshly ground black pepper

1. Preheat the oven to 400°F. Line a sheet pan with parchment paper.

2. Squeeze as much moisture as you can from the sweet potato and zucchini. Combine them in a bowl with the garlic, onion, and egg. Season to taste with salt and pepper.

3. Form the vegetables into four to six small patties and place on the sheet pan, flattening gently with the palm of your hand.

4. Bake for 20 minutes. Remove the pan from the oven and carefully flip the patties. Bake for another 10 minutes.

5. While the patties are cooking, whisk together the mayonnaise, lime, and chipotle.

6. To serve, drizzle the chipotle mayo over the vegetable fritters and sprinkle with fresh cilantro.

SHAKSHUKA

This North African recipe is typically prepared in a cast-iron skillet, but it works just as well on a sheet pan, and oven roasting brings out the sweetness of the peppers and tomatoes. If you prefer to serve it as an appetizer, simply omit the eggs and serve as a dip with beet or parsnip chips.

SERVES: 4   PREP TIME: 10 minutes   COOK TIME: 55 minutes

4 red and orange bell peppers, sliced in long strips

2 yellow onions, sliced in half circles

1 pint grape tomatoes

2 tablespoons olive oil

1 tablespoon fresh thyme leaves

1 teaspoon cumin seeds, crushed

pinch of red chile flakes

8 eggs

½ cup roughly chopped fresh cilantro

½ cup roughly chopped fresh parsley

sea salt

1. Preheat the oven to 375°F.

2. Combine the peppers, onions, and tomatoes on a sheet pan. Drizzle with the olive oil and then add the thyme, cumin, and red chile flakes. Toss to coat thoroughly. Season with salt.

3. Roast uncovered for 45 minutes, stirring once or twice.

4. Remove the pan from the oven and push the vegetables to the side to make eight small wells. Crack an egg into each well and return to the oven to cook for another 10 minutes, or until the egg whites are set. Sprinkle with the cilantro and parsley.

KUNG PAO CAULIFLOWER

Meat is great, but sometimes the flavors of our favorite dishes actually come from the awesome seasonings we add to them. This roasted cauliflower dish will become your new favorite vegan Chinese takeout.

SERVES: 2   PREP TIME: 10 minutes   COOK TIME: 40 to 45 minutes

1 head cauliflower, broken into florets

¼ cup coconut oil

1 teaspoon minced fresh ginger

1 teaspoon minced fresh garlic

¼ teaspoon red chile flakes

1 tablespoon coconut aminos

1 tablespoon maple syrup

1 tablespoon black vinegar or balsamic vinegar

¼ cup toasted cashews

1 scallion, sliced

sea salt

1. Preheat the oven to 375°F. Toss the cauliflower with the coconut oil, ginger, garlic, and red chile flakes. Season with salt. Roast uncovered for 35 to 40 minutes, or until the cauliflower is browned and slightly wilted.

2. Meanwhile, whisk together the coconut aminos, maple syrup, and vinegar. Pour the mixture over the roasted cauliflower and toss with the cashews and scallions. Roast for another 5 minutes.

VEGAN

MUSHROOM AND BOK CHOY BAKE

Mushrooms are perhaps the most suitable meat replacement for veg-etarians because they're real food—which is more than I can say for Frankensoy products—and they're chock-full of healthful vitamins, min-erals, and antioxidants.

SERVES: 2   PREP TIME: 10 minutes   COOK TIME: 25 to 30 minutes

8 ounces cremini or button mushrooms, halved

16 ounces portobello mushrooms, sliced in ½-inch pieces

4 baby bok choy, quartered lengthwise

2 tablespoons coconut oil

1 tablespoon toasted sesame oil

2 tablespoons rice wine vinegar

1 tablespoon minced fresh ginger

2 garlic cloves, minced

sea salt

2 tablespoons sesame seeds

1 scallion, sliced

1. Preheat the oven to 350°F. Line a sheet pan with parchment paper.

2. Spread the mushrooms and bok choy out on the sheet pan.

3. In a small bowl, whisk together the coconut oil, sesame oil, vinegar, ginger, and garlic. Season with salt. Pour the mixture over the mush-rooms and bok choy, tossing to coat.

4. Roast uncovered for 25 to 30 minutes, until the mushrooms are soft and caramelized.

5. Sprinkle with sesame seeds and scallions before serving.

NIGHTSHADE-FREE ▪ VEGAN

VEGETABLE SKEWERS WITH JERK SAUCE

I've been making this jerk sauce for about 10 years and just can't get enough. Originally, I found it the Moosewood Cookbook, but over the years I've adapted it to my personal taste and dietary preferences. Serve over white rice or riced cauliflower.

SERVES: 2   PREP TIME: 20 minutes   COOK TIME: 40 minutes

1 shallot, minced

1 teaspoon minced fresh ginger

2 garlic cloves, minced

1 teaspoon fresh thyme leaves

1 tablespoon ground cinnamon

¼ teaspoon ground allspice

¼ teaspoon red chile flakes

¼ cup red wine vinegar

¼ cup coconut oil

1 zucchini

4 to 6 large button mushrooms, quartered

1 red bell pepper

1 green bell pepper

sea salt

1. Preheat the oven to 375°F. Line a sheet pan with parchment paper.

2. Combine the shallot, ginger, garlic, thyme, and spices in a blender with the vinegar and oil. Puree until smooth. Season to taste with salt.

3. Cut the vegetables into 1-inch chunks and thread onto wooden skewers. Coat thoroughly with the jerk sauce. Place the skewers on the sheet pan.

4. Roast uncovered for 40 minutes until the vegetables are soft and gently browned.

MACADAMIA AND MINT STUFFED EGGPLANT

The macadamia nut cheese resembles feta in this Mediterranean-inspired recipe. The nutritional yeast imparts an umami flavor similar to that of cheese, but it may be omitted if you wish.

SERVES: 4   PREP TIME: 15 minutes   COOK TIME: 35 to 40 minutes

2 medium eggplants

olive oil

1 cup macadamia nuts, soaked in water for 1 hour

½ cup water

1 teaspoon nutritional yeast

4 garlic cloves, divided

1 small shallot

¼ cup minced fresh mint

½ cup raisins

zest of 1 lemon

¼ cup roughly chopped fresh parsley

sea salt

freshly ground pepper

1. Preheat the oven to 375°F.

2. Slice the eggplants in half lengthwise. Brush with oil and season with salt. Place cut-side down on the sheet pan and roast uncovered for 20 minutes.

3. Meanwhile, combine the macadamia nuts, water, nutritional yeast, 2 cloves of garlic, the shallot, and a pinch of salt in a blender. Puree until smooth. Pour the mixture through a nut milk bag or a mesh strainer. Try to remove all of the excess moisture from the nut pulp. Reserve the liquid.

4. Place the nut solids in a mixing bowl. Mince the remaining garlic cloves and add them to the bowl along with the mint, raisins, and lemon zest. Season to taste with salt and pepper.

5. Remove the sheet pan from the oven and turn the eggplant right side up. Scoop out some of the flesh and divide the filling mixture between the eggplants. Return the pan to the oven and cook for another 15 to 20 minutes until lightly browned.

SHEET PAN PALEO

6. Drizzle the remaining macadamia nut "milk" over the finished dish and garnish with fresh parsley.

VEGAN

LEEK AND ONION HAND PIES

In England they're called "pasties," and they're the ultimate in culinary cuteness. This version is made with a simple almond flour pastry crust and has a yummy leek and onion filling. You may skip the precooking of the onion to save time, but it increases the depth of flavor and helps keep the pies from getting too soggy.

SERVES: 4 to 6   PREP TIME: 20 minutes   COOK TIME: 40 to 45 minutes

2 tablespoons olive oil

2 yellow onions, halved then sliced in thin half circles

4 cups blanched almond flour

4 tablespoons tapioca flour, divided

¼ cup palm shortening

5 tablespoons ice water

1 teaspoon sea salt

¼ cup balsamic vinegar

2 leeks, white and pale green parts only

¼ cup fresh basil

freshly ground pepper

1. Warm the olive oil in a large skillet over medium heat. Add the onions and a generous pinch of sea salt, and cook for 10 minutes. The goal is to cook the onions down a bit so they lose some of their moisture.

2. While the onions are cooking, combine the almond flour, 2 tablespoons of the tapioca flour, and 1 teaspoon sea salt in your food processor and pulse once or twice. Add the palm shortening and ice water and blend until thoroughly combined. Divide the mixture into 4 to 6 small balls (depending on how many pies you want) and place in the refrigerator.

3. Pour the balsamic vinegar into the skillet with the onions and allow it to reduce by at least half. Stir in the leeks and basil, and remove from the heat. Season with salt and pepper to taste. Toss with the remaining 2 tablespoons of tapioca flour.

4. Preheat the oven to 325°F. Line a sheet pan with parchment paper.

5. Remove the dough from the refrigerator and roll a ball of dough between two sheets of parchment paper until it is a thin circle. Remove the top square of parchment.

6. Place some of the onion filling on the center of the pastry circle, slightly to one side. Pick up the parchment paper to fold the other side over and press the seam together. Carefully transfer the pie to the sheet pan. Repeat with the remaining pastry dough.

7. Bake uncovered for 40 to 45 minutes until the crust is browned.

NIGHTSHADE-FREE

MUSHROOM AND GARLIC PIE

This is a cross between a deep-dish pizza and a single-crust pie. You could top it with whatever flavors of vegetables and herbs you have, but I absolutely love onions, mushrooms, and thyme together.

SERVES: 4 to 6   PREP TIME: 20 minutes   COOK TIME: 40 to 45 minutes

4 cups blanched almond flour

4 tablespoons tapioca flour, divided

1 teaspoon sea salt

5 tablespoons ice water

¼ cup palm shortening

1 large egg

8 ounces cremini mushrooms, sliced

¼ cup roughly chopped fresh parsley

1 tablespoon fresh thyme

1 yellow onion, halved and thinly sliced

4 garlic cloves, minced

2 tablespoons olive oil

sea salt

freshly ground pepper

½ cup toasted pine nuts, roughly chopped

1. Preheat the oven to 350°F. Line a sheet pan with parchment paper so that it comes up the sides.

2. Combine the almond flour, 2 tablespoons of the tapioca flour, and sea salt in a food processor and pulse once or twice. Add the ice water, palm shortening, and egg and blend until thoroughly combined. Press the mixture into the sheet pan with your hands. I find that using the heels of my hands work best. Press it up the sides, just to the top of the pan.

3. Toss the mushrooms, herbs, onions, and garlic with the olive oil. Season with salt and pepper and toss with the remaining 2 tablespoons tapioca flour. Spread the mixture out over the pastry crust. Top with the pine nuts.

4. Roast uncovered for 30 to 45 minutes, until the topping is browned and bubbling.

NIGHTSHADE-FREE

ROSEMARY, ONION, AND POTATO PIE WITH CABERNET BARBECUE SAUCE

I created this pie one evening from leftovers and some rosemary we picked growing in the neighborhood. It was just divine! You can certainly use a prepared Paleo-friendly barbecue sauce, but the Cabernet barbecue sauce is particularly complex and delicious.

SERVES: 4 PREP TIME: 20 minutes COOK TIME: 40 to 45 minutes

4 cups blanched almond flour

2 tablespoons tapioca flour

1 teaspoon sea salt

5 tablespoons ice water

1 large egg

¼ cup palm shortening

1 cup Cabernet Barbecue Sauce (page 248)

4 Yukon gold potatoes, sliced in paper-thin circles

1 yellow onion, sliced in thin rings

2 teaspoons minced rosemary

1 tablespoon olive oil

freshly ground pepper

1. Preheat the oven to 350°F. Line a sheet pan with parchment paper so that it comes up the sides.

2. Combine the almond flour, tapioca flour, and sea salt in your food processor and pulse once or twice. Add the ice water, egg, and palm shortening and blend until thoroughly combined. Press the mixture into the sheet pan with your hands. I find that using the heels of my hands work best. Press it up the sides, just to the top of the pan.

3. Spread the barbecue sauce along the crust. Top with the potatoes, onions, and rosemary. Brush with olive oil and season with salt and pepper. Bake uncovered for 30 minutes until the toppings are browned and bubbling.

NIGHTSHADE-FREE

CHAPTER FOUR
Fish & Seafood

FISH VERA CRUZ

I absolutely love the briny, salty flavors of this classic Spanish seafood dish. The soft, succulent texture of the fish pairs beautifully with the crisp herbed potatoes.

SERVES: 4   PREP TIME: 15 minutes   COOK TIME: 45 minutes

3 to 4 potatoes, diced in ½-inch pieces

¼ cup minced fresh parsley

2 teaspoons minced garlic, divided

2 tablespoons olive oil

¼ cup capers, drained

½ cup green olives, pitted and roughly chopped

4 plum tomatoes, diced

2 tablespoons red wine vinegar

4 (4- to 6-ounce) halibut fillets

sea salt

freshly ground pepper

1. Preheat the oven to 375°F.

2. Combine the potatoes, parsley, 1 teaspoon of the garlic, and olive oil on a sheet pan. Toss gently to combine. Season with a generous pinch of sea salt. Roast for 30 minutes.

3. Meanwhile, combine the remaining garlic with the capers, olives, plum tomatoes, and vinegar in a small bowl.

4. Cut four 12-inch squares parchment paper. Divide the caper and olive mixture between the sheets of parchment. Top each with a piece of fish. Season with salt and pepper. Fold the parchment to form a loose package.

5. Set the packages atop the potatoes and cook for another 15 minutes.

SALMON WITH CAPER AND RAISIN GREMOLATA AND POTATOES

The sweet raisins, grassy parsley, briny capers, and bright lemon zest are a surprising and flavorful combination. Enjoy with a glass of Sauvignon Blanc and a simple side salad.

SERVES: 2   PREP TIME: 10 minutes   COOK TIME: 45 minutes

1 pound Yukon gold potatoes, diced

3 tablespoons olive oil, divided

1 tablespoon raisins

1 tablespoon minced fresh parsley

zest of 1 lemon

1 tablespoon capers, drained

1 small shallot, minced

1 pound wild salmon fillet

1 lemon, halved

sea salt

freshly ground pepper

1. Preheat the oven to 375°F.

2. Toss the potatoes in 2 tablespoons of the olive oil and season generously with salt and pepper. Roast uncovered for 30 minutes.

3. Meanwhile, soak the raisins in hot water until softened. Drain and mince.

4. Combine the raisins, parsley, lemon zest, capers, shallots, and remaining olive oil in a small bowl. Season with salt and pepper.

5. Dry the salmon gently with paper towels. If it has skin, plan to put it skin-side down on the pan.

6. Spread the gremolata on the salmon with your hands.

7. Push the potatoes aside gently and place the salmon and the lemon halves on the sheet pan between them. Bake for 9 to 11 minutes. The salmon is done when it is still dark in the middle but flakes with a fork.

It will continue cooking after being removed from the oven, so be careful not to overcook it.

8. Slice the fish into individual portions and serve with a lemon half.

SALMON WITH ASPARAGUS

It's easy to prep this recipe ahead of time and have dinner on the table in just 15 short minutes. If you eat rice, that makes an excellent side dish.

SERVES: 4   PREP TIME: 10 minutes   COOK TIME: 15 minutes

1 bunch asparagus, trimmed

1 tablespoon olive oil

4 (4- to 6-ounce) salmon fillets

sea salt

freshly ground pepper

1. Preheat the oven to 350°F.

2. Blanche and shock the asparagus by cooking it in boiling water for 3 to 4 minutes or until brilliant green, then plunging it into ice water to stop the cooking process.

3. Divide the asparagus spears among four sheets of parchment paper. Season generously with salt and pepper and then drizzle with olive oil. Top the asparagus with the salmon fillets. Season again with salt and pepper. Fold the parchment into tight packages and place on a sheet pan.

4. Cook for about 15 minutes, or until cooked to your desired level of doneness.

NIGHTSHADE-FREE ▪ LOW-FODMAP

SPICY CHILI-GLAZED SALMON WITH MASHED PLANTAINS AND GARLIC

My husband and I lived in England for the better part of a year, and our neighborhood market sold salmon fillets in convenient baking packets filled with whatever sauce you asked them to add to it. The spicy chile sauce was our favorite. I've created a Paleo-friendly version that works well with salmon or as a yummy dipping sauce for veggie wraps.

SERVES: 2   PREP TIME: 10 minutes   COOK TIME: 40 minutes

2 to 4 ripe black and yellow plantains

2 (6-ounce) salmon fillets

½ cup Sweet Thai Chili Sauce (page 254)

juice of ½ lime

1 teaspoon minced garlic

sea salt

1. Preheat the oven to 375°F.

2. Cut the ends off of the plantains and place them on the sheet pan. Make a slit down the center of each fruit from one end to the other. Bake uncovered for 30 minutes.

3. Place each salmon fillet individually on a square of parchment paper, coat in the chile sauce, and fold the parchment into a tight package.

4. Remove the plantains from the oven and allow to cool momentarily.

5. Place the salmon packages on the sheet pan and bake for 10 minutes.

6. While the salmon cooks, scrape the cooked plantain into a small bowl and stir in the lime juice and garlic. Season with salt. Serve the mashed plantains topped with a salmon fillet.

SLOW-ROASTED SALMON FILLET WITH ASPARAGUS

Before we called them "hacks," an old trick for cooking salmon was to place it in a dishwasher. It was a convenient way to waste a ton of water and make your dishwasher smell like a dockworker. Gross. Nevertheless, the technique utilized the effectiveness of low, moist heat for cooking salmon. Here is a more efficient method.

SERVES: 4 PREP TIME: 5 minutes COOK TIME: 45 minutes to 1 hour

1 whole king salmon fillet (about 2 pounds)

2 tablespoons olive oil, divided

1 bunch asparagus, trimmed

1 lemon, sliced in thin rings

sea salt

freshly ground pepper

1. Preheat the oven to 200°F. Line a sheet pan with parchment paper. Fill a baking dish with water and place it on the bottom rack of the oven.

2. Place the salmon on the center of the sheet pan and coat with 1 tablespoon of the olive oil. Season with salt and pepper.

3. Scatter the asparagus around the sheet pan and toss with the remaining olive oil. Season with salt and pepper. Top the fish and vegetables with the lemon slices.

4. Bake for 45 minutes to 1 hour, until the salmon is cooked through and the asparagus is soft.

NIGHTSHADE-FREE

WHOLE ROASTED SEA BASS WITH LEEKS

Don't be intimidated by whole fish. When cooked with the skin on and bones present, whole roasted fish retains moisture and is infused with flavor. Serve with a simple side salad.

SERVES: 2   PREP TIME: 10 minutes   COOK TIME: 15 to 20 minutes

2 leeks

2 tablespoons olive oil

2 whole sea bass, 1 to 2 pounds total, gutted, cleaned, and scaled

2 tablespoons minced fresh tarragon

2 tablespoons minced shallots

sea salt

freshly ground pepper

1. Preheat the oven to 450°F.

2. Cut the dark green portions from the ends of the leeks and discard them, halve the white and pale green portions lengthwise, and clean thoroughly under cool running water. Place them on the sheet pan and toss with oil. Season generously with salt and pepper. Roast uncovered for 5 to 10 minutes.

3. Meanwhile, season the fish inside and out with salt and pepper. Divide the tarragon and shallots between the fish, stuffing them into the cavities. Place the fish atop the leeks and continue roasting for another 15 to 20 minutes, or until the fish is cooked through.

4. To serve, simply remove the fin bones from the fish's back and belly sides, then make a slice between the head and the body (where the fish's neck would be) and another slice between the tail and the body. Then slide a knife horizontally along the backbone and another vertically along the backbone. This will allow you to remove the belly fillet, then the back fillet. Remove them to a serving platter. Carefully lift the bone cage and discard it. Remove any membranes and bones from the bottom fillets.

NIGHTSHADE-FREE

WHOLE BAKED TROUT WITH LEMON, FENNEL, AND RAINBOW CARROTS

The sweet roasted vegetables and herbs provide a delicious complement to the robust flavor of trout. When purchasing whole fish, look for bright, clear eyes, shiny skin, vibrant flesh, and a pleasant aroma.

SERVES: 2   PREP TIME: 10 minutes   COOK TIME: 50 minutes

1 lemon, thinly sliced

1 fennel bulb, thinly sliced

4 garlic cloves, shaved thin

1 red onion, sliced in rings

1 pound rainbow carrots, halved lengthwise

1 teaspoon minced fresh rosemary

½ cup roughly chopped fresh parsley

2 tablespoons oil

2 whole trout, about 1 to 1½ pounds total, gutted, cleaned, and scaled

½ cup Paleo Béarnaise Sauce (page 257), for serving

sea salt

freshly ground pepper

1. Preheat the oven to 350°F. Line a sheet pan with parchment paper.

2. On the pan combine the lemon, fennel, garlic, onion, carrots, and herbs with the oil. Season generously with salt and pepper.

3. Roast uncovered for 20 minutes.

4. Remove some of the herbs and small vegetable pieces and carefully place them into the fish cavity. Season generously with salt and pepper.

5. Place the fish atop the remaining vegetables and spoon some of the pan juices over the top of the fish.

6. Roast for another 30 minutes, or until the fish is firm and cooked through.

7. To serve, simply remove the fin bones from the fish's back and belly sides, then make a slice between the head and the body (where the fish's neck would be) and another slice between the tail and the body. Then slide a knife horizontally along the backbone and another vertically along the backbone. This will allow you to remove the belly fillet, then the back fillet. Remove them to a serving platter. Carefully lift the bone cage and discard it. Remove any membranes and bones from the bottom fillets.

NIGHTSHADE-FREE

WHOLE RED SNAPPER WITH CHERMOULA

Chermoula is a classic sauce used in North African cooking. It sounds so exotic, but you most likely have all of the ingredients in your pantry already, except perhaps the preserved lemons, which can be eaten whole. Either make your own or purchase them from a specialty market.

SERVES: 2 to 4   PREP TIME: 15 minutes   COOK TIME: 30 to 35 minutes

1 tablespoon ground coriander

1 tablespoon ground cumin

½ teaspoon smoked paprika

½ teaspoon red chile flakes

1 tablespoon minced garlic

1 preserved lemon, minced

½ cup minced fresh parsley

½ cup minced fresh cilantro

juice of 1 lime

2 whole red snapper, about 1 to 2 pounds total, gutted, cleaned, and scaled

1 zucchini, julienned

2 red bell peppers, sliced in thin strips

2 shallots, thinly sliced

2 tablespoons olive oil

1 lemon, cut into wedges, for serving

sea salt

freshly ground pepper

1. Preheat the oven to 425°F. Line a sheet pan with parchment paper.

2. Combine the spices, garlic, preserved lemon, herbs, and lime juice in a wide, shallow dish. Place the fish in the sauce and turn to coat, spreading it on the inside of the fish as well.

3. Place the zucchini, peppers, and shallots on the sheet pan and coat with the oil. Season with salt and pepper. Roast uncovered for 10 minutes.

4. Place the fish atop the vegetables, drizzle the remaining chermoula over the top, and roast for another 20 to 25 minutes, or until the fish is cooked through.

5. Place the whole fish on a serving platter surrounded by the vegetables and a few fresh lemon wedges.

6. To serve, simply remove the fin bones from the fish's back and belly sides, then make a slice between the head and the body (where the fish's neck would be) and another slice between the tail and the body. Then slide a knife horizontally along the backbone and another vertically along the backbone. This will allow you to remove the belly fillet, then the back fillet. Remove them to a serving platter. Carefully lift the bone cage and discard it. Remove any membranes and bones from the bottom fillets.

PROVENCAL COD WITH ROASTED GRAPE TOMATOES

The sweetness of grape tomatoes intensifies when they're roasted and marries beautifully with the olives, garlic, and herbs in this easy recipe inspired by the south of France.

SERVES: 4   PREP TIME: 5 minutes   COOK TIME: 30 to 35 minutes

2 pints grape tomatoes

1 cup assorted olives

8 to 12 garlic cloves, smashed

4 tablespoons olive oil, divided

zest of 1 orange

1 sprig fresh rosemary, leaves only, minced, divided

3 sprigs fresh thyme, leaves only, divided

4 (4- to 6-ounce) cod fillets

sea salt

freshly ground pepper

1. Preheat the oven to 375°F.

2. Combine the tomatoes, olives, garlic, 2 tablespoons of oil, orange zest, and half of the herbs on a sheet pan. Toss gently to combine. Season with salt and pepper. Roast uncovered for 25 minutes.

3. Meanwhile, dry the cod with paper towels and then coat with the remaining 2 tablespoons olive oil and season with the remaining herbs, salt, and pepper. Set the fish atop the tomato mixture and return to the oven for another 5 to 10 minutes, or until the fish is cooked through.

FISH TACOS WITH SWEET POTATOES

I've been making fish tacos for a long time, but this version is my absolute favorite. The addition of onions, sweet potatoes, and a hefty dose of spices elevates them from basic street food to a gourmet experience. I prefer to purchase whole cumin seeds, coriander seeds, and dried chilies and grind them myself, but you can also purchase them preground.

SERVES: 4   PREP TIME: 10 minutes   COOK TIME: 15 minutes

1 yellow onion

1 large sweet potato

1½ pounds cod, cut into 2-inch pieces

2 tablespoons olive oil

1 tablespoon ground cumin

1 teaspoon ground coriander

1 tablespoon good-quality chili powder

sea salt

16 savoy cabbage leaves, for serving

1 cup Pico de Gallo (page 250), for serving

2 avocados, sliced, for serving

½ cup Cilantro Crema (page 253)

1. Preheat the oven to 375°F. Slice the onion in half vertically and then into thin half circles. Peel the sweet potato and cut into ¼-inch dice. Place the vegetables on the sheet pan along with the cod pieces. Drizzle with oil and toss gently to coat. Season with the spices and a generous pinch of salt and toss gently to coat.

2. Roast uncovered for 15 minutes.

3. To serve, top each cabbage leaf with a portion of fish and vegetables, then top with salsa, avocado, and the cilantro crema.

CRAB-STUFFED SALMON WITH ROASTED CELERIAC, MINT, AND PEAR

One of my first grown-up restaurant experiences was at the original McCormick & Schmick's in downtown Portland, Oregon, where I enjoyed king salmon stuffed with shrimp, crab, and brie cheese. It was so memorable that well over 10 years later, I'm eager to eat it again. This Paleo version swaps the dairy and bread crumbs in the stuffing for pear, mint, and ground macadamia nuts.

SERVES: 4   PREP TIME: 15 minutes   COOK TIME: 50 minutes

2 pounds peeled celeriac (celery root)

2 tablespoons olive oil

6 ounces lump crabmeat

1 tablespoon minced fresh mint

1 ripe pear, peeled and finely diced

½ cup ground macadamia nuts, divided

4 (6-ounce) salmon fillets

sea salt

freshly ground pepper

1. Preheat the oven to 425°F.

2. Dice the celeriac into ½-inch pieces, toss with the olive oil, and season with salt and pepper. Place on a large square of aluminum foil and fold the sides in to form a loose package. Roast in the foil on a sheet pan for 25 minutes.

3. Meanwhile, combine the crab, mint, pear, and ¼ cup of the ground macadamia nuts in a small mixing bowl. Season with salt and pepper.

4. Slice each salmon fillet lengthwise through the top, almost to each end. Divide the crab mixture among the four fillets. Press the remaining ground nuts onto the tops and sides of the salmon and season with salt and pepper.

5. Remove the celeriac from the oven and spread out the foil toward the edges of the sheet pan, pushing the celeriac aside to make space for the salmon fillets. Place the salmon on the foil, which should still have residual oil from the celeriac, and place it in the center of the sheet pan. Return to the oven for 15 minutes or until the salmon is barely opaque in the center.

NIGHTSHADE-FREE

MEDITERRANEAN SALMON EN PAPILLOTE

For a native Northwesterner who knows how exquisite perfectly cooked salmon can be, preparing it at home can be an intimidating task. One minute it's underdone, and the next minute it can be tough as jerky. The secret to creating the sunset pink–hued interior that flakes under gentle pressure is even, moist heat, which is created by cooking each fillet in its own parchment envelope.

SERVES: 2   PREP TIME: 10 minutes   COOK TIME: 15 minutes

1 zucchini, julienned

1 yellow bell pepper, sliced into thin spears

1 tablespoons olive oil

1 tablespoon balsamic vinegar

¼ cup fresh basil, cut into thin pieces

2 (4- to 6-ounce) salmon fillets

sea salt

freshly ground pepper

1. Preheat the oven to 325°F.

2. Combine the zucchini and bell pepper in a small bowl and toss with the oil and vinegar. Add the basil. Divide the mixture between two large squares of parchment paper. Season with salt and pepper.

3. Place a salmon fillet on top of each mound of vegetables and season with salt and pepper.

4. Pull the opposite sides of the parchment paper up so that they meet in the middle. Fold them down together, as if folding a paper lunch sack, until you reach the fish. Then tuck each end under. Place on the sheet pan and roast for 15 minutes or until the fish is cooked through.

AHI TUNA AND MUSHROOM BAKE

Prepared medium rare, ahi tuna is a real delicacy, so make sure you buy sushi-grade fish from a quality purveyor. You might think "fresh" tuna is the best option, but when fish is flash-frozen after it's caught and remains that way until you thaw it for cooking, it will retain quality and be safer to consume at rare or medium-rare temperatures.

SERVES: 2   PREP TIME: 5 minutes   COOK TIME: 15 minutes

8 ounces cremini or button mushrooms, halved

3 tablespoons toasted sesame oil, divided

1 tablespoon minced garlic

zest and juice of 1 lime

1 tablespoon minced fresh ginger

1 pound ahi tuna, cut into 1½-inch pieces

4 cups salad greens

handful fresh cilantro, roughly chopped

sea salt

freshly ground pepper

1. Preheat the oven to 400°F.

2. Place the mushrooms on a sheet pan and toss with 2 tablespoons of the sesame oil and the garlic, and season with salt and pepper. Roast for 10 minutes.

3. Meanwhile, whisk together the remaining 1 tablespoon sesame oil, lime juice, and ginger in a large bowl. Add the tuna and gently turn to coat. Season with salt and pepper.

4. Add the fish to the sheet pan, tossing gently with the mushrooms, and continue cooking for another 5 minutes.

5. To serve, divide the salad greens and cilantro between two plates and top with the mushrooms and tuna, drizzling any pan juices over the greens.

NIGHTSHADE-FREE

PROSCIUTTO-WRAPPED SCALLOPS WITH ROASTED APPLES

The flavors of pork, scallops, and apples marry beautifully in this simple oven-roasted dinner. It's lovely on its own or served over mixed baby greens.

SERVES: 2 to 4   PREP TIME: 15 minutes   COOK TIME: 30 to 35 minutes

3 to 4 Pink Lady apples, peeled and cored

1 tablespoon coconut oil

1 tablespoon sherry vinegar

1 teaspoon ground cinnamon

2 ounces sliced prosciutto

1 pound large sea scallops

sea salt

freshly ground pepper

1. Preheat the oven to 400°F.

2. Cut the apples into 8 wedges each. In a large bowl, whisk together the oil, vinegar, and cinnamon. Toss the apples in the mixture to coat. Spread out on a sheet pan. Season with salt. Bake for 20 minutes.

3. Meanwhile, slice the prosciutto lengthwise. Pat the scallops dry with a paper towel. Wrap each scallop in one slice of prosciutto. Season the scallops generously with salt and pepper.

4. Push the apple slices aside to make room for the scallops on the sheet pan. Roast for 10 to 15 minutes, or until the scallops are cooked through.

NIGHTSHADE-FREE

ROCK SALT-ROASTED PRAWNS AND FINGERLING POTATOES

Salt conducts heat beautifully for a moist, flavorful shrimp and buttery potatoes.

SERVES: 2   PREP TIME: 5 minutes   COOK TIME: 48 minutes

3 to 4 pounds rock salt

1 pound fingerling potatoes

1 pound large prawns, unpeeled

1 lemon, cut into wedges

salad greens, for serving

1. Preheat the oven to 400°F.

2. Spread half of the rock salt onto a rimmed sheet pan. Add the potatoes and cover with the remaining rock salt. They may not be completely submerged, but that's okay.

3. Roast for 40 minutes. Carefully remove the pan from the oven and carve out several spaces in the salt for the prawns, then cover them by gently spooning salt over the top.

4. Return to the oven and roast for another 8 minutes. Check one of the prawns to test for doneness.

5. Remove the pan from the oven and allow to rest for 10 minutes before brushing the salt off.

6. Serve with simple salad greens and a squeeze of lemon juice.

LOW-FODMAP

HALIBUT WITH CAULIFLOWER, GARLIC, AND CARAMELIZED FENNEL

This dish was a happy accident that occurred when I was trying to use up vegetables before they withered. But what a pleasant surprise it was to bite into the crispy, caramelized fennel dripping in olive oil and lemon juice. Although the ingredients are few, the preparation is what really transforms them!

SERVES: 2   PREP TIME: 10 minutes   COOK TIME: 27 to 35 minutes

1 head cauliflower

1 fennel bulb

2 garlic cloves, very finely minced

2 to 4 tablespoons olive oil

2 (4- to 6-ounce) halibut fillets

juice of 1 lemon

sea salt

freshly ground pepper

1. Preheat the oven to 375°F.

2. Break the cauliflower into florets, cutting the larger ones in half. Quarter, core, and slice the fennel bulb into very thin slices. Place the vegetables on the sheet pan. Toss with the garlic and olive oil, then season generously with salt and pepper.

3. Roast for 20 to 25 minutes uncovered. Remove from the oven and toss gently to brown on the other side. Make spaces in the vegetables and place the halibut fillets. Season with salt and pepper and about half of the lemon juice.

4. Roast for another 7 to 10 minutes, depending on the thickness of the halibut and your desired level of doneness.

5. Squeeze the remaining lemon juice over the halibut and vegetables and serve.

NIGHTSHADE-FREE

SPANISH SHRIMP AND SPINACH

This dish is a riff on the classic Spanish tapas with spinach and chick-peas, but trades the legumes for a Paleo-friendly protein. It is lovely as an appetizer or served over Sweet Potato Oven Fries (page 18) for a complete meal.

SERVES: 2 to 4   PREP TIME: 5 minutes   COOK TIME: 12 minutes

2 tablespoons olive oil

2 garlic cloves, minced

⅛ teaspoon red chile flakes

1 tablespoon smoked paprika

1 tablespoon ground cumin

pinch of sea salt

1 pound peeled, deveined large shrimp, at least 20/26 per pound

2 plum tomatoes, diced

2 bunches fresh spinach, thoroughly rinsed

2 tablespoons red wine vinegar

1. Preheat the oven to 375°F.

2. Whisk together the oil, garlic, and spices in a medium bowl. Add a generous pinch of salt. Toss the shrimp in the mixture to coat thoroughly. Spread the shrimp out on the sheet pan along with the diced tomatoes and roast uncovered for 10 minutes.

3. Add the spinach to the sheet pan, tossing gently with the shrimp to combine. Return the pan to the oven for 2 minutes.

4. Drizzle the red wine vinegar over the mixture and toss to combine.

BAKED CLAMS WITH CAPERS, TOMATOES, AND BASIL

The flavors of capers, tomatoes, and fresh basil make a perfect backdrop for fresh clams. If the ones at the market don't look and smell awesome, mussels or prawns will work equally well. If you prefer to use fresh plum tomatoes, blanch and shock them, then peel the skins off before using in this recipe.

SERVES: 2   PREP TIME: 10 minutes   COOK TIME: 30 minutes

1 (28-ounce) can plum tomatoes, drained, hand torn

¼ cup capers, drained, roughly chopped

4 to 6 garlic cloves, smashed

1 yellow onion, sliced in very thin rings

1 cup fresh basil, hand torn, divided

1 tablespoon fennel seed, ground

pinch of red chile flakes

pinch of sea salt

½ cup dry white wine

1 to 2 pounds fresh clams, scrubbed

1. Preheat the oven to 350°F.

2. Spread the tomatoes, capers, garlic, onion, and half of the basil out on a sheet pan. Drizzle with olive oil and season with the ground fennel, chile flakes, and a pinch of sea salt. Pour the white wine over the mixture.

3. Bake uncovered for 20 minutes. Remove the pan from the oven and nestle the clams into the mixture, ladling some of the vegetables over the shells.

4. Return the pan to the oven and bake until the clams open, about 10 more minutes. Shower with the remaining fresh basil.

BROILED OYSTERS WITH LEMON AND ZUCCHINI

Oysters are the superstar of seafood when it comes to nutrient density. They're an amazing source of vitamin B12, zinc, selenium, and copper. Paired with a zucchini "pasta," this dish is a refreshing summer dinner.

SERVES: 2   PREP TIME: 20 minutes   COOK TIME: 2 minutes

2 zucchini

pinch of sea salt

1 dozen oysters

1 tablespoon olive oil

2 lemons

1 shallot, minced

¼ cup roughly chopped fresh parsley

freshly ground pepper

1. Cut the zucchini into noodles with a spiralizer, or use a mandoline or vegetable peeler to achieve long, thin strands that resemble spaghetti. Toss the noodles with a generous pinch of salt and set in a colander to sweat out some of their moisture.

2. Scrub and rinse the oysters thoroughly using a vegetable brush. One at a time, place them in a dish towel and use an oyster knife to pry the shells apart. Be careful not to damage the meat or pour the juice out. Slide the knife beneath the meat to dislodge it from the shell. Repeat with the remaining oysters.

3. Preheat the broiler to high and place the oven rack on the top shelf.

4. Zest and juice one of the lemons. Rinse and wring the zucchini noodles of excess moisture. Toss them with the olive oil, lemon juice, and lemon zest on the sheet pan. Nestle the oyster halves into the noodles. Top with the minced shallot. Broil for 2 minutes.

5. Sprinkle with the parsley and season with salt and pepper.

6. Slice the remaining lemon into wedges and serve them with the oysters and zucchini noodles.

NIGHTSHADE-FREE

LOBSTER TAILS WITH BABY RED POTATOES AND HERBS

Lobster enjoys a reputation as the king of crustaceans, making it intimidating for everyday dinners. But don't let its rock star status keep you away. It's loaded with nutrients and tastes pretty good too. Serve it simply with potatoes and fresh herbs.

SERVES: 2 to 4   PREP TIME: 5 minutes   COOK TIME: 25 to 30 minutes

1 pound baby red potatoes

2 tablespoons olive oil, divided

2 lobster tails

sea salt

freshly ground pepper

2 tablespoons fresh minced chives

2 tablespoons fresh minced parsley

1 lemon, halved

1. Preheat the oven to 375°F.

2. Spread the potatoes out on the sheet pan and drizzle with 1 tablespoon of the olive oil.

3. Cut the lobster tails in half lengthwise. Using a pair of scissors, cut and remove the cartilage covering the tail meat from the shell. Place the tails on the sheet pan between the potatoes. Season everything with salt and pepper. Roast uncovered for 25 to 30 minutes, or until the lobster meat is firm and opaque.

4. Shower with the fresh herbs and drizzle with lemon juice just before serving.

LOW-FODMAP

BASIC CRAB CAKES WITH STEAMED ASPARAGUS

Most crab cakes rely on bread crumbs as a binder, which is a bummer for grain-free folks. Fortunately, the sheet pan answers the problem beautifully and allows the cakes to hold together without bread. When they are baked, you get a moist, firm cake that's gently browned.

SERVES: 2 to 4   PREP TIME: 10 minutes   COOK TIME: 25 minutes

½ cup Paleo Mayonnaise (page 251) or a store-bought Paleo-friendly mayo

1 egg white, beaten

2 garlic cloves, minced

1 scallion, minced

1 teaspoon gluten-free Worcestershire sauce, such as Lea & Perrins

1½ teaspoons Old Bay Seasoning

1 pound lump crabmeat

1 bunch asparagus, trimmed

1 tablespoon olive oil

zest and juice of 1 lemon

sea salt

freshly ground pepper

1. Preheat the oven to 400°F. Line a sheet pan with parchment paper.

2. Whisk together the mayonnaise, egg white, garlic, scallion, Worcestershire sauce, and Old Bay Seasoning. Fold in the crabmeat gently until all of the ingredients are thoroughly integrated without breaking up the pieces of crab. Season with salt.

3. Form the mixture into six 1-inch-thick cakes and place on the sheet pan.

4. Place the asparagus on a sheet of parchment and season with the olive oil, lemon zest, salt, and pepper, and then fold the parchment into a package to allow the asparagus a moist environment in which to cook. Place it on the sheet pan.

5. Bake the crab cakes and asparagus for 15 minutes. Flip the cakes and cook for another 10 minutes until browned and set.

6. Squeeze the lemon juice over the crab cakes and asparagus.

SPICY ASIAN CRAB CAKES

SERVES: 2 to 4   PREP TIME: 10 minutes   COOK TIME: 25 minutes

½ cup Paleo Mayonnaise (page 251) or a store-bought Paleo-friendly mayo

1 egg white, beaten

1 tablespoon minced fresh ginger

2 garlic cloves, minced

1 scallion, minced

1 tablespoon hot sauce

1 pound lump crabmeat

sea salt

1 lime, cut into wedges for serving

4 cups mixed greens, for serving

½ cup Cilantro Crema (page 253)

1. Preheat the oven to 400°F. Line a sheet pan with parchment paper.

2. Whisk together the mayonnaise, egg white, ginger, garlic, scallion, and hot sauce. Fold in the crabmeat gently until all of the ingredients are thoroughly integrated without breaking up the pieces of crab. Season with salt.

3. Form the mixture into six 1-inch-thick cakes and place on the sheet pan.

4. Bake uncovered for 15 minutes. Flip the cakes and cook for another 10 minutes until browned and set.

5. Serve with lime wedges, mixed greens, and cilantro crema.

SALMON CAKES AND POTATO SKINS

I have been making this same recipe for nearly a decade now. But I've been cooking the salmon cakes on the stovetop to varying degrees of success. Because I don't use nonstick pans, sometimes the cakes stick to the pan and I lose the delicious brown crust. Who knew that in writing this book I would discover the secret to perfect salmon cakes? The sheet pan is the absolute best way to cook these.

SERVES: 2   PREP TIME: 15 minutes   COOK TIME: 1 hour

3 small to medium Russet potatoes, scrubbed

1 shallot, minced

¼ cup minced fresh cilantro

1 egg, whisked

1 (16-ounce) can cooked salmon

2 tablespoons olive oil

sea salt

freshly ground pepper

1. Preheat the oven to 400°F. Pierce the potatoes with a fork several times. Bake for 35 to 40 minutes. Remove from the oven and slice into quarters lengthwise. Allow to cool briefly and then scoop the inner flesh of the potato from the skins.

2. Meanwhile, combine the shallot, cilantro, and egg in a mixing bowl. Mash the cooked potato flesh with the back of a fork and stir it into the egg mixture until thoroughly integrated. Fold in the salmon and stir until just combined. Season with salt and pepper.

3. Line a sheet pan with parchment paper. Form the salmon mixture into 6 or 8 cakes about 1-inch-thick and place them on one end of the sheet pan. Lay the potato skins on the other end of the pan and brush them with olive oil and then season with salt and pepper.

4. Bake for 20 minutes, flipping the salmon cakes about halfway through the cooking, until browned and set.

ROSEMARY SCALLOP KEBABS WITH CHORIZO AND ROASTED SWEET POTATOES

The rosemary and chorizo infuse the scallops with flavor. Paired with sweet potatoes, this makes a deliciously satisfying meal. It pairs well with a dry Spanish sherry.

SERVES: 4   PREP TIME: 15 minutes   COOK TIME: 40 minutes

3 to 4 sweet potatoes, diced

2 tablespoons olive oil

6 to 8 rosemary sprigs

1½ pounds large sea scallops

4 ounces Spanish chorizo, thinly sliced

1 lemon, cut into wedges

sea salt

freshly ground pepper

1. Preheat the oven to 375°F.

2. Spread the sweet potatoes out on a sheet pan. Mince the needles from one of the rosemary sprigs and add it to the pan and toss with the olive oil and sweet potatoes. Season with salt and pepper. Roast uncovered for 25 minutes.

3. Meanwhile, thread the scallops and chorizo slices onto remaining rosemary skewers beginning at the bottom of the stem, alternating between the two ingredients. Set them on top of the sweet potatoes and roast for another 15 to 20 minutes. Roasting time will depend on the size of the scallops and thickness of the chorizo slices.

4. Serve with lemon wedges.

WHOLE SHRIMP WITH BACON AND COLLARDS

Bacon and collard greens not only taste amazing together, but it's also a pretty healthy combination. The fat in the bacon helps your body absorb the vitamins and minerals in the collards. Throw in some whole shrimp and you have Paleo meal perfection.

SERVES: 2 to 4   PREP TIME: 15 minutes   COOK TIME: 30 to 35 minutes

juice of 1 lemon

2 tablespoons olive oil

1 tablespoon minced garlic, divided

2 pounds whole jumbo shrimp, peeled and deveined

2 ounces applewood-smoked bacon, diced

1 bunch collard greens, tough ribs removed

sea salt

freshly ground pepper

1. Combine the lemon juice, olive oil, and 2 teaspoons of the minced garlic in a mixing bowl. Toss the shrimp in the mixture to coat thoroughly. Set aside. This step can be done up to 2 hours in advance to enhance the flavor of the shrimp.

2. Preheat the oven to 400°F. Line a sheet pan with parchment paper.

3. In a small skillet, cook the bacon over medium-low heat until it renders most of its fat.

4. Meanwhile, roll the entire bunch of collard greens in a tight cylinder and make a chiffonade by cutting the roll crosswise into thin ribbons.

5. Place the greens on the sheet pan and top with the bacon pieces and bacon fat. Add the remaining minced garlic. Toss gently to combine. Top with the marinated shrimp.

6. Roast uncovered for 10 to 15 minutes, or until the shrimp is cooked through and the collards are wilted.

NIGHTSHADE-FREE

CHAPTER FIVE
Poultry

PLANTAIN-CRUSTED CHICKEN TENDERLOINS WITH STEAMED CARROTS

This kid-friendly recipe has the delightful crunch of breaded chicken pieces, but they are made with ground plantain chips. Find them in the bulk section of your health food market or online, and look for chips that have been cooked in coconut or palm oil.

SERVES: 2   PREP TIME: 10 minutes   COOK TIME: 30 minutes

2 carrots, cut into spears

1 teaspoon olive oil

1 10- to 12-ounce boneless skinless chicken breast, cut into long strips

1 egg, whisked

½ cup ground plantain chips

sea salt

freshly ground pepper

1. Preheat the oven to 350°F. Place the carrots on a large square of aluminum foil. Drizzle with olive oil and sprinkle with salt. Toss gently to coat. Fold the foil into a tight pouch and place on a sheet pan. Bake for 10 minutes.

2. Meanwhile, pat the chicken piece dry. Place the ground plantain chips in a shallow dish and season with salt and pepper, stirring to combine.

3. Drench the chicken in the egg, then dredge in the ground plantains.

4. Remove the pan from the oven and add the coated chicken pieces. Bake for another 10 minutes, turn the chicken over, and bake for 10 minutes until the chicken is cooked through.

NIGHTSHADE-FREE · LOW-FODMAP

SALSA VERDE ROASTED CHICKEN BREASTS

Cooking the chicken in salsa verde keeps it beautifully moist. Enjoy on its own or over white rice or sweet potato fries.

SERVES: 4   PREP TIME: 5 minutes   COOK TIME: 30 to 40 minutes

4 10- to 12-ounce boneless skinless chicken breasts

1 yellow onion, sliced in thick rings

4 cups salsa verde

½ cup roughly chopped fresh cilantro

sea salt

freshly ground pepper

1. Preheat the oven to 350°F.

2. Place the chicken breasts between two sheets of parchment paper and pound to a uniform thickness. Place it on a sheet pan and scatter the onions around it. Season with salt and pepper.

3. Pour the salsa verde into the pan and turn the chicken and onions to coat.

4. Roast uncovered for 30 to 40 minutes, or until the chicken is cooked to an internal temperature of 165°F.

5. To serve, top with fresh cilantro.

CHILLED CRISPY CHICKEN AND VEGETABLES

The flavors of the vegetables in this dish are mesmerizing, and the chicken skin stays magically crisp. It's perfect for a hot summer dinner or a picnic lunch.

SERVES: 4   PREP TIME: 10 minutes   COOK TIME: 45 minutes

2 zucchini

4 small beets, with 1-inch stems

4 carrots

3 to 4 shallots, halved lengthwise

2 tablespoons fresh thyme leaves

olive oil

2 bone-in 12- to 14-ounce chicken breasts

2 tablespoons red wine vinegar

sea salt

freshly ground pepper

1. Preheat the oven to 425°F.

2. Slice the zucchini into 1-inch rounds. Slice the beets in half lengthwise. Cut the carrots in half both vertically and horizontally, so each one yields 4 pieces. Toss the vegetables, including the shallots, on the sheet pan with the thyme and a moderate drizzle of olive oil. Season with salt and pepper.

3. Dry the chicken breasts thoroughly and then coat them in olive oil. Season with salt and pepper. Place on the sheet pan between the vegetables.

4. Roast uncovered for 45 minutes, or until the vegetables are very tender and caramelized and the chicken has reached an internal temperature of 160°F. (It will continue cooking after being removed from the oven.)

5. Toss with the red wine vinegar and refrigerate until ready to serve.

NIGHTSHADE-FREE

ROASTED CHICKEN WITH BACON-GLAZED BRUSSELS SPROUTS AND CARAMELIZED ONIONS

This is the kind of dish you would order in a restaurant and then return to the restaurant just to order it again. And again. It's that good.

SERVES: 2 to 4   PREP TIME: 15 minutes   COOK TIME: 45 minutes

⅓ cup rendered bacon fat, melted

½ yellow onion, diced

1 teaspoon sherry vinegar

2 teaspoons maple syrup, divided

1 pound Brussels sprouts, rinsed, outer leaves removed, and halved

1 whole chicken (3 to 4 pounds)

sea salt

freshly ground pepper

1. Preheat the oven to 375°F.

2. Heat 1 tablespoon of bacon fat in a large skillet over medium-low heat. Cook the onions with a pinch of salt until soft, about 10 minutes. Add the sherry vinegar and 1 teaspoon of the maple syrup. Cook for another 5 minutes.

3. Meanwhile, spread the Brussels sprouts out on a sheet pan. Coat with 2 tablespoons of the bacon grease and season generously with salt and pepper. Top with the caramelized onions.

4. Lay the chicken out on a cutting board breast-side down. Using a sharp knife or a pair of kitchen shears, cut down each side of the backbone. Remove it and save for another use, such as making stock.

5. Season the cut-side of the chicken with salt and pepper. Place it cut-side down on the sheet pan pushing the Brussels sprouts to the sides. Thoroughly dry the chicken skin with paper towels and then pour the remaining bacon fat over it, rubbing with your fingers to coat thoroughly. Season generously with salt and pepper.

7. Roast uncovered for 30 minutes. Remove the vegetables to a heat-proof bowl and drizzle with the remaining 1 tablespoon maple syrup. Cover tightly with foil to keep warm.

8. Return the chicken to the oven and roast until cooked through to an internal temperature of 165°F, about another 15 minutes. Allow it to rest for 5 minutes before cutting into pieces. Serve with the Brussels sprouts.

NIGHTSHADE-FREE

PESTO CHICKEN WITH GRAPE TOMATOES

Although you could purchase a prepared pesto from your local market, most varieties contain Parmesan cheese and often industrial oils. If you're sensitive to dairy or simply choose to avoid it, this quick and easy version is equally delicious. Use a dry skillet to toast the pine nuts until fragrant for a more complex flavor.

SERVES: 4   PREP TIME: 10 minutes   COOK TIME: 30 to 40 minutes

¼ cup olive oil

1 cup loosely packed fresh basil

¼ cup toasted pine nuts

zest of 1 lemon

generous pinch of sea salt

4 to 6 boneless, skinless chicken thighs

1 pint grape tomatoes

1. Preheat the oven to 400°F.

2. Combine the oil, basil, pine nuts, lemon zest, and salt in a blender. Puree until mostly smooth.

3. Place the chicken on a baking sheet and pour the pesto over. Toss to coat. Add the tomatoes.

4. Bake uncovered for 30 to 40 minutes, or until the chicken is cooked through to an internal temperature of 165F.

LOW-FODMAP

ROASTED CHICKEN THIGHS WITH WINTER VEGETABLES

I enjoyed this amazing dish for the first time a few days before Christmas while visiting my friend Anna in Colorado. The weather was bitter-cold outside, which made this succulent combination of crispy chicken and caramelized vegetables particularly comforting. We enjoyed it with our shared favorite Trader Joe's red wine, Cocobon.

SERVES: 2 to 4   PREP TIME: 10 minutes   COOK TIME: 55 minutes

½ kabocha squash

1 large parsnip

6 rainbow carrots

1 red onion

¼ cup plus 2 tablespoons coconut oil, melted

4 to 6 bone-in, skin-on chicken thighs

sea salt

freshly ground pepper

1. Preheat the oven to 400°F. Line a baking sheet with parchment paper.

2. Slice the kabocha into ¼- to ½-inch half circles. Cut the parsnips, carrots, and onion into 2-inch chunks.

3. Toss the vegetables with ¼ cup of the coconut oil and a generous pinch of sea salt and place them on the baking sheet. Bake uncovered for 10 to 15 minutes.

4. Meanwhile, pat the chicken thighs dry with a paper towel and heat the remaining 2 tablespoons coconut oil in a wide skillet over medium-high heat. Season the meat generously with salt and pepper. Cook skin-side down for 3 to 4 minutes, turn over, and cook for another 3 minutes.

5. After the thighs are browned, place them skin-side up on top of the roasting veggies and continue to roast it all for another 30 to 40 minutes until cooked to an internal temperature of 165°F.

SAUSAGE, FENNEL, AND CHICKEN DRUMSTICKS

This chicken drumstick recipe strikes the perfect balance between ease of preparation and depth of flavor with fewer than five ingredients! As it cooks, the fennel caramelizes and produces a soft, creamy texture that complements the savory Italian sausage and chicken legs beautifully.

SERVES: 2   PREP TIME: 10 minutes   COOK TIME: 40 to 45 minutes

2 fennel bulbs

4 hot Italian sausages

8 chicken drumsticks

1/4 cup olive oil

freshly ground pepper

sea salt

1. Preheat the oven to 375°F.

2. Slice the fennel bulbs into quarters and then into ½-inch-thick pieces. If you wish to leave the base of the bulb intact, it will keep each of the slices held together, but it is too tough to be palatable.

3. Slice the sausage in 1- to 2-inch-long pieces.

4. Arrange the fennel, chicken, and sausage on a sheet pan.

5. Drizzle with olive oil, tossing to coat. Season with salt and pepper.

6. Bake for 40 to 45 minutes, or until the chicken is cooked through to an internal temperature of 165°F and the fennel is soft. If the chicken and sausage cook more quickly, you may remove it to a serving platter and continue cooking the fennel for another 10 minutes.

BACON-SKINNED CHICKEN BREAST WITH ROSEMARY FINGERLING POTATOES

One spring, my kids and I cleared a plot in the community garden for a new gardener. We transplanted plenty of sunflowers and picked kale for dinner, but the biggest surprise—or the smallest actually—was the multitude of tiny gold potatoes we unearthed. We roasted them in a bit of olive oil with fresh rosemary alongside split chicken breast for dinner that night, and my oldest remarked, "I can't believe we just picked these today!" I just love those little opportunities to introduce the kids to fresh vegetables. Assuming you don't have a bed of potatoes waiting in your garden, choose fingerling potatoes or another small, golden potato for this recipe.

SERVES: 2 to 4   PREP TIME: 10 minutes   COOK TIME: 45 minutes

1 pound fingerling potatoes, scrubbed

2 tablespoons olive oil

1 sprig fresh rosemary, needles minced

2 bone-in, skin-on chicken breasts

4 bacon slices, preferably applewood smoked

sea salt

freshly ground pepper

1. Preheat the oven to 400°F.

2. Toss the potatoes with the oil and rosemary on the sheet pan. Season generously with salt.

3. Slide your fingers between the chicken skin and meat to separate them. Place the bacon slices under the skin. Season the underside of the breasts with salt and pepper. Dry the skin side thoroughly with a paper towel. Place the meat on the sheet pan, pushing the potatoes aside to make space.

4. Roast the chicken and potatoes for 45 minutes, or until the chicken is cooked through to an internal temperature of 165°F.

CORNISH GAME HENS WITH MUSHROOMS AND WILTED KALE

This is perfect for late winter when you just want warm comfort food with minimal fuss. I'm partial to cooking with my oven in the winter because it heats the whole house so beautifully. Enjoy with a glass of earthy red wine, such as Sangiovese, a good book, and a cozy fire.

SERVES: 2   PREP TIME: 10 minutes   COOK TIME: 30 minutes

8 ounces cremini mushrooms, quartered

2 to 3 tablespoons ghee or coconut oil

2 Cornish game hens, backbones removed and flattened

6 to 8 leaves Lacinato kale

2 tablespoons olive oil

2 garlic cloves, finely minced

2 teaspoons red wine vinegar

sea salt

freshly ground pepper

1. Preheat the oven to 375°F.

2. Toss the mushrooms in most of the ghee or oil. Spread around the sheet pan, making space for the hens. Season generously with salt and pepper.

3. Place the game hens on the sheet pan and coat with the remaining ghee or oil. Season generously with salt and pepper.

4. Bake uncovered for 20 to 30 minutes, or until the hens are cooked through to an internal temperature of 165°F.

5. Meanwhile, remove the kale ribs, roll the leaves in at tight cylinder, and make a chiffonade by cutting the roll crosswise into thin ribbons. Toss with the olive oil and garlic.

6. When the game hens are cooked, remove them to a cutting board to rest. Add the kale to the sheet pan with the mushrooms and cook for 8 to 10 minutes until wilted. Season the kale and mushrooms with the red wine vinegar and salt and pepper to taste.

NIGHTSHADE-FREE

ROASTED CHICKEN MOLE WITH BAKED SWEET POTATOES

Serve this flavorful chicken with small roasted sweet potatoes cooked directly on the oven rack. The prep time for the sauce is long, but it's well worth the effort!

SERVES: 4 to 6   PREP TIME: 30 minutes   COOK TIME: 45 minutes

3 cups Quick Paleo Mole (page 246), divided

6 to 8 bone-in chicken thighs

4 to 6 small sweet potatoes, scrubbed and pierced with a fork

1. Preheat the oven to 325°F.

2. Pour the mole onto a sheet pan, reserving about 1 cup. Place the chicken thighs on the pan and then cover with the remaining sauce. Cover the pan tightly with foil.

3. Place the pan on the top rack of the oven for 45 minutes, or until the chicken is cooked through to an internal temperature of 165°F. Roast the sweet potatoes on the bottom rack of the oven.

4. About halfway through the cooking time, remove the foil from the pan.

5. To serve, slice each sweet potato lengthwise and top with a piece of chicken and a generous spoonful of sauce.

CHICKEN FAJITAS

Cabbage leaves are my favorite tortilla alternative. However, if you have a hankering for something that more closely resembles a flour tortilla, you can purchase grain-free wraps online or make your own.

SERVES: 4   PREP TIME: 10 minutes   COOK TIME: 30 minutes

1 yellow onion, halved

1 red bell pepper, sliced

1 green bell pepper, sliced

1 yellow bell pepper, sliced

4 cloves garlic, thinly sliced

2 pounds boneless, skinless chicken breasts, cut into 2-inch strips

¼ teaspoon cayenne pepper

1 teaspoon smoked paprika

1 teaspoon ground cumin

½ teaspoon sea salt

2 tablespoons olive oil

8 to 12 cabbage leaves, for serving

1 lime, cut into wedges

1 avocado, sliced

handful fresh cilantro, for serving

1. Preheat the oven to 375°F. Line a sheet pan with parchment paper

2. Spread the vegetables and chicken pieces out on the sheet pan.

3. In a small measuring cup, whisk together the spices, salt, and oil. Pour the mixture over the chicken and vegetables, turning to coat.

4. Roast uncovered for 30 minutes, or until the chicken is cooked through to an internal temperature of 165°F and the vegetables are browned and soft.

5. Serve the fajita mixture in cabbage leaves and top with a squeeze of lime juice, a slice of avocado, and a few sprigs of cilantro.

WHITE WINE BRAISED CHICKEN

While living in Europe, I fell in love with French cooking. Beef bourguignon and coq au vin blanc were two of my favorite recipes. Although coq au vin is traditionally made with red wine, I prefer the color and flavor of white wine. It's worth the extra effort to brown the chicken pieces before cooking in the oven, but if you're short on time, you may omit this step.

SERVES: 4   PREP TIME: 20 minutes   COOK TIME: 45 to 50 minutes

4 ounces pancetta, diced

1 cup pearl onions, peeled (frozen and thawed is okay)

1 cup cremini mushrooms, quartered

8 carrots with 1-inch of green tops remaining

1 tablespoon fresh thyme leaves

1 whole chicken about 3 to 4 pounds total, cut into pieces

1 to 2 cups dry white wine

sea salt

freshly ground pepper

1. Preheat the oven to 375°F.

2. Cook the pancetta in a large skillet over medium heat until the fat is rendered, about 10 minutes.

3. Spread the onions, mushrooms, and carrots out on a rimmed sheet pan. Add the thyme and season with salt and pepper.

4. Remove the cooked pancetta from the pan and sprinkle it over the vegetables.

5. Turn the heat up to medium-high. Season the chicken on both sides with salt and pepper. Brown it in the rendered pancetta fat for 2 to 3 minutes on each side. You may have to do this in batches. Place the chicken skin-side up in among the vegetables. Pour any remaining oil onto the vegetables.

6. Transfer the pan to the oven and then carefully add the wine so that it comes up the sides of the chicken but does not overflow the pan.

7. Roast uncovered for 45 to 50 minutes, or until the chicken is cooked to an internal temperature of 165°F. Allow to rest for 10 minutes before removing the chicken and vegetables to a serving platter.

NIGHTSHADE-FREE

FILIPINO ADOBO CHICKEN WITH BUTTERNUT SQUASH

Traditionally, adobo chicken needs no accompaniment other than rice. But for a one-pan meal, butternut squash is a lovely grain-free alternative and it's loaded with nutrients. Also, traditional adobo chicken is marinated in soy sauce, but because soy is generally avoided on a Paleo diet, I've used fish sauce instead.

SERVES: 4   PREP TIME: 15 minutes, plus 12 hours for marinating   COOK TIME: 25 to 30 minutes

¼ cup fish sauce

¼ cup rice wine vinegar

2 tablespoons maple syrup

1 tablespoon minced fresh ginger

6 to 8 garlic cloves, smashed

2 serrano chiles, thinly sliced

½ cup coconut oil, divided

8 bone-in, skin-on chicken thighs

1 butternut squash, peeled and cut into 1-inch cubes

sea salt

freshly ground pepper

1. Combine the fish sauce, vinegar, maple syrup, ginger, garlic, and chiles in a nonreactive bowl. Season with salt and pepper. Whisk in all but 2 tablespoons of the coconut oil. Add the chicken thighs and coat thoroughly with the marinade. Cover and refrigerate for 12 hours.

2. Preheat the oven to 450°F. Line a sheet pan with parchment paper.

3. Toss the butternut squash with the remaining coconut oil and season with salt and pepper. Spread it out on the sheet pan.

4. Remove the chicken thighs from the marinade and place them skin-side up on the sheet pan. Roast uncovered for 25 to 30 minutes, or until the chicken reaches an internal temperature of 165°F.

CHICKEN TIKKA MASALA

To the Indian food purists out there, I'm sorry. I realize oven roasting isn't a traditional method for making tikka masala. But, if you want amazing Indian flavors with just one pan, you're in for a treat.

SERVES: 4   PREP TIME: 10 minutes   COOK TIME: 25 to 30 minutes

4 boneless, bone-in, chicken breast halves, skin removed

1 tablespoon coconut oil

1 onion, halved then sliced in thin rings

1 tablespoon ground coriander

1 tablespoon smoked paprika

1 ½ teaspoons ground cumin

½ teaspoon ground cardamom

¼ teaspoon cayenne pepper

1 tablespoon grated fresh ginger

1 (15-ounce) can tomato puree

1 (15-ounce) can coconut milk

1 teaspoon sea salt

½ cup roughly chopped fresh cilantro

1. Preheat the oven to 375°F. Line a sheet pan with parchment paper.

2. Pound the chicken breasts between two sheets of parchment paper until they are uniformly ½ inch thick. Coat them in coconut oil and place them on the sheet pan. Top with the onion slices.

3. In a medium mixing bowl, whisk together the spices, ginger, tomato puree, coconut milk, and salt. Pour the mixture over the chicken and onions, turning to coat.

4. Roast uncovered for 25 to 30 minutes, or until the chicken is cooked through to an internal temperature of 165°F. Garnish with the cilantro.

LEMON-GARLIC CHICKEN WITH WILTED SPINACH

I thought there were only so many ways to serve chicken and vege-tables—that is, until I stumbled upon this recipe. It offers a bright and surprising combination of flavors and textures.

SERVES: 2 to 4   PREP TIME: 10 minutes   COOK TIME: 45 minutes

2 tablespoons olive oil

zest of 1 lemon

2 garlic cloves, minced

1 teaspoon minced fresh rosemary

2 bone-in, skin-on chicken breasts, about 12- to 14-ounces

2 bunches fresh spinach, thoroughly rinsed and dried

½ teaspoon ground allspice

½ teaspoon ground coriander

¼ teaspoon ground cinnamon

1. Preheat the oven to 425°F.

2. Whisk together the olive oil, lemon zest, garlic, and rosemary. Rub it onto the chicken breasts and place them onto a sheet pan.

3. Roast the chicken uncovered for 40 to 45 minutes, or until cooked to an internal temperature of 165°F.

4. When the chicken has finished cooking, remove it to a cutting board to rest.

5. Place the spinach and spices on the sheet pan and toss to coat in the pan juices. Return to the oven for 1 to 2 minutes, or until the spinach is just wilted but before it has released too much moisture.

BUTTERNUT SQUASH CASSOULET

This traditional French stew contains cannellini beans, salt pork, sausage, and chicken or duck. Fortunately, you can achieve all of the same flavors without the beans. I've used butternut squash in their place, but feel free to substitute another starchy vegetable.

SERVES: 4   PREP TIME: 10 minutes   COOK TIME: 1 hour 12 minutes

4 ounces pancetta, diced

1 butternut squash, peeled and diced

1 yellow onion, diced

2 celery stalks, diced

2 carrots, diced

4 garlic cloves, smashed

½ to 1 cup chicken broth

1 ½ pounds bone-in, skin-on chicken pieces (thighs, wings, and drumsticks)

2 garlic sausages, cut into 2-inch pieces

1 tablespoon olive oil

sea salt

freshly ground pepper

1. Preheat the oven to 375°F.

2. Combine the pancetta, squash, onion, celery, carrots, and garlic on a rimmed sheet pan. Season with salt and pepper. Pour in the chicken broth so it comes partially up the sides of the pan.

3. Top the vegetables with the chicken and sausage. Brush with olive oil and season with salt and pepper.

4. Cover tightly with aluminum foil. Roast for 45 minutes.

5. Remove the foil and continue cooking for another 25 minutes or until the chicken is cooked through to an internal temperature of 165°F.

6. Finish the dish by cooking under the broiler for 2 to 3 minutes to brown the chicken.

TURKEY BREAST STUFFED WITH LEEKS AND DATES

The presentation of this stuffed turkey breast is beautiful enough for holiday gatherings. Although it requires a bit of advance preparation, it's worth the effort! I've used escarole as a vegetable side, but you could also swap it out for radicchio or endive.

SERVES: 4 to 6   PREP TIME: 25 minutes   COOK TIME: 20 minutes

4 ounces pancetta

2 leeks, white and pale green parts only, halved lengthwise and rinsed thoroughly

1 whole turkey breast, about 3 pounds, cut from the bone

4 medjool dates, roughly chopped

2 tablespoons olive oil, divided

1 bunch escarole, hand torn

sea salt

freshly ground pepper

1. Cook the pancetta over medium heat in a large skillet until it has rendered its fat, about 10 minutes. Remove to a separate dish.

2. Place the leeks in the skillet and cook in the rendered fat until lightly browned and soft, about 10 minutes.

3. Preheat the oven to 400°F. Line a sheet pan with parchment paper.

4. While the leeks are cooking, butterfly the turkey breast by cutting through it horizontally until it is nearly sliced into two large pieces. Fold it open so that the meat lays flat on the cutting board, skin-side down. Lay the cooked leeks on one side of the meat, top with the chopped dates, and season the whole thing with salt and pepper. Roll the meat as if rolling up a rug so that the filling is neatly tucked inside. You may wish to tie the whole thing together with kitchen twine.

5. Rub the outside of the turkey with 1 tablespoon of the olive oil and season with salt and pepper. Place in the center of the sheet pan.

6. Scatter escarole around the turkey and drizzle with the remaining olive oil, season with salt and pepper, and sprinkle with the cooked pancetta.

7. Roast uncovered for 20 minutes, stirring the escarole once. The meat should reach an internal temperature of 160°F.

WHOLE ROASTED TURKEY

One year, my husband and I spent Thanksgiving morning at the beach surfing with friends. We arrived at home to a 12-pound bird sitting in the refrigerator and only two hours before our guests arrived. Fortunately, I had just discovered the beauty of the spatchcock method for roasting chicken, and decided to give it a try for the turkey. While it didn't offer that Norman Rockwell appearance, the bird was beautifully browned and fully cooked just in time for dinner.

SERVES: 4 to 6   PREP TIME: 10 minutes, plus 12 hours for brining   COOK TIME: 2 hours

1 cup sea salt	2 cinnamon sticks
½ cup peppercorns	2 cups boiling water
½ cup coconut palm sugar	1 gallon ice-cold water
2 bay leaves	1 whole turkey (12 to 15 pounds)
2 tablespoons allspice berries	¼ cup rendered bacon fat

1. Combine the salt, peppercorns, palm sugar, bay leaves, allspice berries, and cinnamon sticks in the boiling water and allow to dissolve. Add it to the ice-cold water and place the turkey in the brine overnight. If you do not have space for it in your refrigerator, top the turkey with a few pounds of crushed ice and replace as needed to keep the water temperature below 40°F.

2. Preheat the oven to 450°F.

3. Remove the turkey from the brine and pat dry thoroughly with paper towels. Remove the backbone from the turkey by placing it breast-side down on a cutting board. Using sharp kitchen shears, cut down one side of the backbone and then the other. Remove it and save for making stock or another use. Flatten the bird with the heel of your hand.

4. Rub the turkey with the rendered bacon fat on all sides and place cut-side down on the sheet pan. Roast uncovered for 15 minutes, then reduce the heat to 325°F and continue roasting for 10 to 15 minutes per pound of meat until the bird reaches an internal temperature of 165°F in the deepest part of the breast.

5. Allow to rest for 15 minutes before slicing and serving.

ROAST TURKEY LEGS WITH BRUSSELS SPROUTS

I've heard these called "caveman pops," which is fitting for Paleo dieters. The dark turkey meat is loaded with nutrients and offers a much better portion size, in my mind, than skimpy chicken legs. In keeping with turkey's association with Thanksgiving, I've paired them with Brussels sprouts.

SERVES: 4　PREP TIME: 10 minutes　COOK TIME: 90 minutes

4 turkey legs

3 tablespoons rendered bacon fat

1½ pounds Brussels sprouts

4 cloves garlic, smashed

sea salt

freshly ground pepper

1. Preheat the oven to 350°F. Line a sheet pan with parchment paper and place an oven-safe rack over it.

2. Coat the turkey legs in 2 tablespoons of the rendered bacon fat and season with salt and pepper. Place them on the rack and roast for 45 minutes.

3. Meanwhile, halve the Brussels sprouts and remove any discolored outer leaves. Toss them with the remaining bacon fat and garlic cloves. Carefully remove the rack from the sheet pan and add the sprouts to the bottom of the pan, tossing to coat with the turkey drippings. Season with salt and pepper.

4. Return the rack to the pan, turn the turkey legs over, and return the pan to the oven to roast for another 45 minutes, or until the turkey reaches an internal temperature of 180°F.

NIGHTSHADE-FREE

SPICY TURKEY LEGS WITH SWEET POTATOES

If you want a delicious meal that will keep you full for hours, try these spicy turkey legs. They're loaded with protein, fat, and safe starch to keep you satisfied. Look for a brand of chipotles in adobo, such as Roland, that does not contain wheat flour, soybean oil, or high-fructose corn syrup.

SERVES: 4 PREP TIME: 10 minutes COOK TIME: 90 minutes

3 tablespoons rendered bacon fat, divided

2 chipotles in adobo sauce, finely chopped, plus 2 tablespoons adobo sauce

4 turkey legs

4 sweet potatoes, unpeeled, diced

1 yellow onion, halved then sliced thinly

4 garlic cloves, roughly chopped

sea salt

freshly ground pepper

1. Preheat the oven to 350°F. Line a sheet pan with parchment paper and place an oven-safe rack over it.

2. Whisk together 2 tablespoons of the bacon fat and adobo sauce, and coat the turkey legs in this mixture. Season with salt and pepper. Place them on the rack and roast for 45 minutes.

3. Meanwhile, toss the sweet potatoes, onion, and garlic with the remaining bacon fat and chipotles. Carefully remove the rack from the sheet pan and add the vegetables to the bottom of the pan, tossing to coat with the turkey drippings. Season with salt and pepper.

4. Return the rack to the pan, turn the turkey legs over, and return the pan to the oven to roast for another 45 minutes or until the turkey reaches an internal temperature of 180°F.

MIDDLE EASTERN TURKEY MEATBALL WRAPS

In the Paleo community, fear of saturated fat is a thing of the past, leading many of us to overlook ground turkey as a replacement for beef. But turkey has twice the potassium of ground beef, making it a healthy alternative.

SERVES: 2   PREP TIME: 10 minutes   COOK TIME: 15 to 20 minutes

1 pound ground turkey

2 tablespoons flax meal

1 egg

1 tablespoon minced garlic, divided

1 shallot, minced

1 teaspoon dried oregano

½ teaspoon sea salt

½ teaspoon ground pepper

½ cup tahini

juice of 1 lemon

leaves of 1 head butter lettuce, for serving

½ cup parsley

1 cup grape tomatoes, halved

1. Preheat the oven to 375°F. Place an oven-safe rack on top of a sheet pan.

2. Use your hands to combine the turkey, flax meal, egg, 2 teaspoons of the garlic, shallots, oregano, salt, and pepper in a large bowl. Form the mixture into 8 balls and place on the sheet pan. Bake uncovered for 15 to 20 minutes, or until cooked to an internal temperature of 165°F. Allow the meatballs to rest for 10 minutes before serving.

3. While the meatballs are cooking, whisk together the tahini, remaining 1 teaspoon garlic, and lemon juice, and season with salt and pepper.

4. To serve, place two meatballs in a lettuce leaf and top with fresh parsley, a few tomatoes, and a generous drizzle of tahini sauce.

BARBECUE TURKEY MEATBALLS

It doesn't get any better than a giant pan full of meatballs slathered in a tangy barbecue sauce. My favorite pairing for the sauce is a simple coleslaw, which is delicious served on top. You can use the simple barbecue sauce recipe below or purchase a Paleo-friendly sauce, which are becoming more widely available in health food stores and online.

SERVES: 4   PREP TIME: 10 minutes   COOK TIME: 25 to 30 minutes

2 pounds ground turkey

¼ cup flax meal

2 eggs

1 teaspoon minced garlic

1 shallot, minced

1 teaspoon smoked paprika

¼ teaspoon cayenne pepper

1 teaspoon sea salt

½ teaspoon freshly ground pepper

For the Barbecue Sauce:

1 (15-ounce) can tomato sauce

2 tablespoons coconut palm sugar

1 tablespoon smoked paprika

½ teaspoon cayenne pepper

1 tablespoon Dijon mustard

¼ cup apple cider vinegar

1. Preheat the oven to 375°F.

2. Use your hands to combine the turkey, flax meal, eggs, garlic, shallots, paprika, cayenne, salt, and pepper in a large bowl. Form the mixture into 12 to 16 large balls and place on the sheet pan. Bake uncovered for 15 minutes.

3. Meanwhile, whisk together the barbecue sauce ingredients in a small bowl. Pour it over the meatballs and cook for another 10 to 15 minutes, or until the meatballs are cooked to an internal temperature of 165°F. Allow the meatballs to rest for 10 minutes before serving.

BROILED DUCK BREAST WITH PLUM SAUCE OVER SHAVED FENNEL AND BABY GREENS

Duck pairs beautifully with sweet sauces. This one is made with dried plums, which is code for prunes. But don't worry, they're actually quite decadent, especially when served alongside a delicate and bright salad.

SERVES: 4   PREP TIME: 10 minutes   COOK TIME: 30 minutes

4 Muscovy duck breasts

1 dozen dried plums

2 sprigs fresh thyme

1 cup fruity red wine, such as Zinfandel

sea salt

freshly ground pepper

2 tablespoons olive oil

1 tablespoon champagne vinegar or white wine vinegar

½ fennel bulb, cored and thinly sliced

8 cups mixed baby greens

1. Preheat the broiler. Place the oven rack near the top of the oven, so the pan will be about 5 inches from the element.

2. Place the plums, thyme, and red wine on a sheet pan.

3. Score the duck skin in a diamond pattern at 1-inch intervals. You want to cut through the skin and fat but not into the meat. Season both sides of the meat with salt and pepper.

4. Place the duck breast skin-side down on the rack. Broil for 7 minutes. Turn the duck breast over and broil for another 7 minutes, or until the duck reaches an internal temperature of 130°F for medium rare. Allow to rest on a cutting board for 5 minutes before serving.

5. Carefully pour the plums and wine into a blender. Discard the thyme sprigs. Puree until smooth. Season to taste.

6. Whisk together the olive oil and vinegar, and toss with the fennel and greens to coat. Place some on the center of each plate.

7. To serve, slice the duck on a bias and place it over each salad. Drizzle with the plum sauce. Serve immediately.

NIGHTSHADE-FREE

BROILED DUCK BREAST WITH BELGIAN ENDIVE

Typically, duck breast is seared on the stovetop to render fat from under the skin, and then it's finished in the oven. Fortunately, you can accomplish this effect entirely in the oven using your broiler.

SERVES: 4   PREP TIME: 10 minutes   COOK TIME: 30 minutes

6 Belgian endive, halved lengthwise

2 tablespoons olive oil

4 Muscovy duck breasts

2 tablespoons balsamic vinegar reduction or good-quality balsamic vinegar

sea salt

freshly ground pepper

1. Preheat the oven to 400°F. Line a sheet pan with parchment paper. Place the oven rack near the top of the oven, so the pan will be about 5 inches from the heating element.

2. Toss the endive with olive oil and season with salt and pepper. Place them cut-side up on the sheet pan. Roast uncovered for 15 minutes. Remove the pan from the oven, turn the endive over and top the pan with an oven-safe rack.

3. Preheat the broiler.

4. Score the duck skin in a diamond pattern at 1-inch intervals. You want to cut through the skin and fat but not into the meat. Season both sides of the meat with salt and pepper.

5. Place the duck breast skin-side down on the rack. Broil for 7 minutes. Turn the duck breast over and broil for another 7 minutes, or until the duck reaches an internal temperature of 130°F for medium rare. Allow to rest for 5 minutes before serving.

6. Toss the endive with the balsamic vinegar.

7. To serve, slice the duck on a bias and top with a spoonful of the pan juices and serve with the endive.

NIGHTSHADE-FREE

DUCK LEGS WITH AROMATIC VEGETABLES

There's something decidedly elegant about duck legs, so I've paired them with classic French vegetables and herbs. You can certainly vary the vegetables according to what you have on hand, substituting onions for leeks and whatever woody herbs are available.

SERVES: 4   PREP TIME: 10 minutes   COOK TIME: 1 hour and 5 minutes

4 duck legs

2 leeks, white and pale green parts only, thinly sliced in circles

4 carrots, diced

6 garlic cloves, roughly chopped

leaves of 4 sprigs thyme

1 cup chicken or vegetable broth

½ cup dry white wine

sea salt

freshly ground pepper

1. Preheat the broiler and place the oven rack at the top about five inches from the heating element. Season the duck legs with salt and pepper and place them skin-side up on the sheet pan. Broil for 5 minutes. Remove the pan from the oven and turn the oven temperature to bake at 350°F.

2. Scatter the leeks, carrots, and garlic around the duck legs, sprinkle with the thyme, season with salt and pepper, and pour in the wine. Add the chicken or vegetable broth until it comes halfway up the sides of the pan.

3. Return the pan to the oven and roast for 1 hour, or until the duck reaches an internal temperature of 170°F.

NIGHTSHADE-FREE

ASIAN-SPICED DUCK LEGS OVER SAVOY CABBAGE SLAW

The Chinese five-spice powder and ginger pair beautifully with fatty duck legs in this recipe. A tangy, crunchy salad offers the perfect backdrop and a nice textural contrast.

SERVES: 4   PREP TIME: 10 minutes   COOK TIME: 1 hour

4 duck legs

1 teaspoon minced fresh ginger

1 teaspoon Chinese five-spice powder

4 cups shredded savoy cabbage

1 green onion, thinly sliced on a bias

½ cup roughly chopped fresh cilantro

1 tablespoon toasted sesame oil

1 teaspoon honey

1 tablespoon rice wine vinegar

1 teaspoon Chinese mustard

sea salt

freshly ground pepper

1. Preheat the oven to 375°F. Season the duck legs with the ginger, five-spice powder, and salt and pepper, and place them skin-side up on the sheet pan. Roast uncovered for 1 hour, or until the duck reaches an internal temperature of 170°F.

2. Meanwhile, toss the cabbage, onions, and cilantro together in a large bowl. Whisk together the sesame oil, honey, vinegar, and mustard. Drizzle it over the fresh greens just before serving.

3. Allow the duck to rest for 10 minutes before slicing and serving over the salad greens.

HERB-ROASTED DUCK LEGS WITH WINTER VEGETABLES

When you're craving comfort food, look no further than roasted vegetables and duck leg. The herbs elevate these ingredients from everyday to absolutely sublime.

SERVES: 4   PREP TIME: 10 minutes   COOK TIME: 1 hour

4 duck legs

1 tablespoon fresh thyme leaves

1 tablespoon minced fresh rosemary

1 tablespoon minced fresh parsley

1 yellow onion, sliced in rings

4 parsnips, sliced in 3-inch pieces

4 turnips, quartered

2 tablespoons olive oil

sea salt

freshly ground pepper

1. Preheat the oven to 375°F. Line a sheet pan with parchment paper.

2. Season the duck legs with the herbs, salt, and pepper, and place them skin-side up on the sheet pan. Toss the vegetables with the olive oil and season with salt and pepper. Place them around the duck legs.

3. Roast uncovered for 1 hour, or until the duck reaches an internal temperature of 170°F. Stir the vegetables once or twice during the cooking process to cook them evenly.

4. Allow the duck to rest for 10 minutes before serving with the vegetables.

NIGHTSHADE-FREE

DUCK CONFIT WITH BLANCHED GREEN BEANS AND FRISEE

One of my favorite things about following a Paleo-style of eating is that I'm no longer afraid of dietary fat. This classic preparation for duck requires very little accompaniment. I'm partial to a cold salad of blanched green beans and frisee drenched in fresh lemon juice.

SERVES: 4   PREP TIME: 10 minutes   COOK TIME: 2 to 3 hours

6 to 8 duck pieces (breasts and legs)

1 tablespoon herbes de Provence

1 shallot, minced

2 garlic cloves, minced

4 cups duck fat

1 pound blanched green beans

4 cups frisee

juice of 1 lemon

sea salt

freshly ground pepper

1. Preheat the oven to 325°F. Line a sheet pan with parchment paper.

2. Place the duck pieces in a single layer on the sheet pan and season with the herbes de Provence, shallots, garlic, salt, and pepper.

3. Melt the duck fat and pour it over the duck pieces.

4. Roast uncovered for 2 to 3 hours, or until the duck is quite tender. Remove it to a platter and allow to cool. Toss the green beans and frisee with lemon juice and season with salt and pepper. Serve with the duck confit.

NIGHTSHADE-FREE

CHAPTER SIX

Pork

FIVE-SPICE PORK SIRLOIN ROAST WITH RADICCHIO AND PEAR SAUCE

This recipe has all the warmth, sweetness, and spice you look for in a holiday dinner. If you're comfortable eating dairy, add a few table-spoons of softened butter or ghee to the pear sauce for an extra layer of decadence.

SERVES: 4 to 6   PREP TIME: 15 minutes, plus 4 to 6 hours for brining   COOK TIME: 50 to 60 minutes

1½ tablespoons Chinese five-spice powder, divided

2 tablespoons red wine vinegar

2 tablespoons maple syrup or coconut palm sugar

2 tablespoons sea salt

½ cup hot water

2 cups ice water, or more as needed

1 boneless pork sirloin roast (2 to 3 pounds)

3 tablespoons olive oil, divided

1 head radicchio, sliced in wedges

¼ cup balsamic vinegar

2 tablespoons olive oil, divided

2 pears, unpeeled, cored and sliced in wedges

2 tablespoons butter or ghee (optional)

1. Combine 1 tablespoon of the Chinese five-spice powder with the red wine vinegar, maple syrup or palm sugar, and salt in a deep, nonreactive deep dish. Add the hot water and whisk to combine. Add the ice water. Submerge the pork roast in the brine, adding more ice water as needed to cover. Refrigerate for 4 to 6 hours.

2. Preheat the oven to 350°F. Line a sheet pan with parchment paper.

3. Remove the pork roast from the brine and pat dry with paper towels. Coat with 1 tablespoon of the oil to facilitate browning. Roast uncovered for 25 to 30 minutes per pound of meat (e.g., for a 2-pound roast, cooking time would be 50 to 60 minutes).

4. During the last 30 minutes of cooking, whisk together the balsamic vinegar, remaining 2 tablespoons oil, and remaining ½ tablespoon five-spice powder. Dredge the radicchio slices in the vinegar mixture and scatter across the sheet pan along with the pear slices. Return to the oven and roast uncovered until the pork is cooked through to an internal temperature of 145°F.

5. Remove the pork to a cutting board and cover with foil for 10 minutes before slicing.

6. Place the pears in a blender along with any pan juices and puree until smooth. Add the butter or ghee if using to further thicken the sauce.

7. Slice the meat on a bias and serve with the pear sauce and radicchio.

ROASTED PORK TENDERLOIN WITH SPICED PLUMS AND CARAMELIZED ONIONS

Roasted plums really could be in the dessert chapter, but they're just so exquisite next to roast pork tenderloin, I couldn't help myself. They're also a pretty classic accompaniment for roast pork.

SERVES: 4 to 6   PREP TIME: 10 minutes   COOK TIME: 50 to 60 minutes

1 boneless pork sirloin roast (2 to 3 pounds)

3 tablespoons olive oil, divided

6 plums, halved and pitted

1 teaspoon ground cinnamon

¼ teaspoon freshly grated nutmeg

1 red onion, sliced in thin rings

1. Preheat the oven to 350°F. Line a sheet pan with parchment paper.

2. Pat the pork loin dry with paper towels. Coat with 1 tablespoon of the oil to facilitate browning.

3. Toss the plums with 1 tablespoon of the olive oil and the cinnamon and nutmeg. Spread them out on the sheet pan. Coat the onion slices in the 1 tablespoon remaining oil and add them to the sheet pan. Season the whole pan generously with salt and pepper.

4. Roast uncovered for 25 to 30 minutes per pound of meat until the meat reaches an internal temperature of 145°F (e.g., for a 2-pound roast, cooking time would be 50 to 60 minutes).

5. Remove the pork to a cutting board and cover with foil for 10 minutes before slicing.

PORK TENDERLOIN STUFFED WITH SHALLOTS, ROSEMARY, AND PEARS

Infuse the pork with flavor from the inside out with this sweet and savory stuffing. It's delicious with roasted parsnips, but you could also use turnips for a little spice.

SERVES: 4 to 6   PREP TIME: 10 minutes   COOK TIME: 50 to 60 minutes

1 boneless pork sirloin roast (2 to 3 pounds)

2 shallots, minced

1 pear, peeled and diced

2 sprigs rosemary, minced

3 tablespoons olive oil, divided

6 parsnips, unpeeled, halved lengthwise

sea salt

freshly ground pepper

1. Preheat the oven to 450°F. Line a sheet pan with parchment paper.

2. Pat the pork loin dry with paper towels. Slice it down the center lengthwise nearly all the way through.

3. Place the shallots, pear, and half of the rosemary in the center of the pork loin, season with salt and pepper, and then close the meat back up, tying with kitchen twine.

4. Coat the exterior of the pork with about half of the olive oil to facilitate browning. Season the outside with sea salt and freshly ground pepper. Set on the center of the sheet pan.

5. Toss the parsnips with the remaining olive oil and rosemary and season with salt. Place on the sheet pan around the pork loin.

6. Roast uncovered for 25 to 30 minutes per pound of meat (e.g., for a 2-pound roast, cooking time would be 50 to 60 minutes).

7. Remove the pork to a cutting board and cover with foil for 10 minutes before slicing.

CORIANDER AND FENNEL SPICED BABYBACK PORK RIBS

Whole fennel and coriander seeds ground and rubbed into pork ribs impart a complex and flavorful crust to the meat's exterior. A sweet and savory peach and onion compote provides a luscious textural contrast.

SERVES: 2   PREP TIME: 15 minutes, plus 1 to 24 hours for marinating
COOK TIME: 1½ hours

1 tablespoon whole coriander seeds

1 teaspoon whole fennel seeds

½ teaspoon red chile flakes

1 teaspoon sea salt

2 tablespoons coconut palm sugar

2 babyback rib racks, about 1½ to 2 pounds total

2 garlic cloves, minced

¼ cup dry white wine

2 yellow onions, thinly sliced

2 ripe peaches, thinly sliced

1 tablespoon fresh thyme leaves

2 tablespoons rendered bacon fat or olive oil

sea salt

freshly ground pepper

1. Grind the coriander, fennel, and red chile flakes in a spice grinder until coarsely ground. Add the salt and palm sugar and pulse until thoroughly combined. Rub the mixture over the rib racks and wrap them individually in parchment paper to form tight packages. Refrigerate for at least 1 hour or up to 24 hours.

2. Preheat the oven to 300°F. Place the ribs in their parchment packages on a sheet pan. Divide the garlic and white wine between the packages, folding to reseal, and roast for 30 minutes.

3. Meanwhile combine the onions, peaches, thyme, and bacon fat or olive oil on a large square of parchment paper. Season with salt and pepper. Fold it into a tight package and place on the sheet pan along with the rib racks. Roast for another hour.

4. During the final 30 minutes of cooking, remove everything from its parchment and spread out on the sheet pan to finish cooking or until the meat reaches an internal temperature of 145°F.

5. Allow the meat to rest for 10 minutes or more before slicing and serving with the onions and peaches.

BARBECUE PORK RIBS

Sometimes you just don't want to fire up the grill but you crave the smoky flavors of food hot off the flames. These roasted pork ribs coated in a smoked paprika dry rub will satisfy your cravings. Enjoy them with coleslaw and whole roasted sweet potatoes for a delicious summer meal.

SERVES: 4   PREP TIME: 10 minutes   COOK TIME: 1½ to 2 hours

3 to 4 pounds baby back ribs

2 tablespoons coconut oil

¼ cup smoked paprika

1 tablespoon dry mustard

½ teaspoon cayenne pepper

1 tablespoon coconut palm sugar

1 teaspoon sea salt

2 cups Barbecue Sauce (page 245), or use a quality store-bought Paleo-friendly sauce

1. Place an oven safe rack on a sheet pan. Set the pork ribs on top of the rack and coat with coconut oil. In a small mixing bowl, combine the spices, sugar, and salt. Rub the mixture into the ribs and set them on the rack meaty-side up. Or, to intensify the flavor, place the ribs in the refrigerator for several hours to allow the flavors to permeate the meat.

2. Preheat the broiler to high and position a rack a few inches from the heating element. Broil the ribs for 5 minutes. Move the pan to the middle rack and roast at 300°F for 1½ to 2 hours or until the meat reaches an internal temperature of 145°F.

3. During the last 15 minutes of cooking, pour a cup of barbecue sauce over the pork ribs and continue roasting.

4. Serve with the remaining barbecue sauce.

PORK CHOPS WITH APPLES AND ONIONS

Bone-in meats remain blissfully moist when cooked, although they take slightly longer to cook than their boneless counterparts. This recipe for bone-in pork chops is perfect for a weeknight supper—simply prep the apples and onions before you leave for work in the morning and your dinner is half done!

SERVES: 4   PREP TIME: 10 minutes   COOK TIME: 30 to 35 minutes

4 tart apples

2 yellow onions

2 tablespoons coconut oil, divided

4 bone-in pork chops, about 8 ounces each

sea salt

freshly ground pepper

1. Preheat the oven to 400°F.

2. Core the apples and slice into ¼-inch wedges. Slice the onions into ¼-inch rings. Combine them with 1 tablespoon of the coconut oil on a sheet pan. Toss to coat. Roast uncovered for 15 minutes.

3. Rub the pork chops with the remaining 1 tablespoon coconut oil. Season with salt and pepper. Remove the sheet pan from the oven and push the onions and apples aside to make space for the pork chops. Return the pan to the oven for 15 to 20 minutes, or until the chops register an internal temperature between 140° and 145°F.

NIGHTSHADE-FREE

PEPPER-BRINED PORK CHOPS WITH RADICCHIO AND PORT REDUCTION

These pork chops get a double dose of spice from a peppery brine and a generous seasoning before they go into the oven. Cut the spice with a sweet port reduction.

SERVES: 4 PREP TIME: 20 minutes, plus up to 8 hours for brining COOK TIME: 10 minutes

1 cup water

¼ cup multicolored peppercorns

1 tablespoon coconut palm sugar

1 tablespoon sea salt

1 garlic clove, smashed

2 tablespoons red wine vinegar

2 cups ice

4 bone-in pork chops, about 8 ounces each

4 tablespoons olive oil, divided

4 heads radicchio, halved lengthwise

½ cup Port Reduction (page 256)

sea salt

freshly ground pepper

1. Bring of the water to a simmer in a saucepan with the peppercorns, palm sugar, sea salt, and garlic, stirring until the salt and sugar are dissolved. Stir in the vinegar. Cool the mixture by adding the ice. Brine the meat for at least 1 hour and up to 8 hours in a nonreactive dish in the refrigerator.

2. Preheat the oven to 400°F. Line a sheet pan with parchment paper.

3. Place the radicchio cut-side down on the pan and drizzle with two tablespoons of the olive oil, turning a few times to coat. Season with salt and pepper.

4. Remove the pork from the brine and pat dry with paper towels. Coat with the remaining 2 tablespoons olive oil and season generously with pepper. Place alongside the radicchio.

5. Roast uncovered for 15 to 20 minutes, or until the chops register an internal temperature between 140° and 145°F.

6. Drizzle the port reduction over the pork chops to serve.

PORK CHOPS WITH ROASTED GRAPES, SWISS CHARD, AND TOASTED ALMONDS

There's something very satisfying about the tangy sweetness of the roasted grapes and Swiss chard topped with crunchy almonds. Sherry vinegar is a nice touch, but if you don't have any, red wine vinegar works as well.

SERVES: 4   PREP TIME: 10 minutes   COOK TIME: 15 to 20 minutes

2 cups red seedless grapes

2 tablespoons olive oil, divided

4 bone-in pork chops about 8 ounces each

1 bunch Swiss chard, stems and leaves roughly chopped

1 teaspoon sherry vinegar or red wine vinegar

2 tablespoons toasted almonds, roughly chopped

sea salt

freshly ground pepper

1. Preheat the oven to 400°F. Line a sheet pan with parchment paper

2. Spread the grapes on the sheet pan. Roast uncovered for 15 minutes.

3. Rub the pork chops with 1 tablespoon of the olive oil. Season with salt and pepper. Remove the sheet pan from the oven and push the grapes aside to make space for the pork chops. Return the pan to the oven for 15 minutes.

4. Coat the chard stems with the remaining olive oil. Add them to the pan for the final 5 minutes of cooking.

5. Remove the pan from the oven and toss the roasted grapes with the chard leaves and the vinegar in a small bowl. Season with salt and pepper and top with the almonds.

NIGHTSHADE-FREE

PORK CHOPS WITH PEACH CHUTNEY

Inspired by the flavors of India, this simple dish is sweet, sour, and spicy. Enjoy it over steamed white rice or with a simple side salad.

SERVES: 4   PREP TIME: 10 minutes   COOK TIME: 15 to 20 minutes

4 peaches, thinly sliced

1 red bell pepper, thinly sliced

1 red onion, halved and thinly sliced

1 teaspoon curry powder

⅛ teaspoon red chile flakes

1 tablespoon maple syrup

2 tablespoons coconut oil, divided

4 bone-in pork chops, about 8 ounces each

1 tablespoons red wine vinegar

½ cup roughly chopped fresh cilantro

sea salt

freshly ground pepper

1. Preheat the oven to 400°F.

2. Toss the peaches, bell pepper, and onion with the curry powder, red chile flakes, maple syrup, and 1 tablespoon of the coconut oil on a sheet pan. Toss to coat. Season with salt and pepper.

3. Rub the pork chops with the remaining 1 tablespoon coconut oil. Season with salt and pepper. Roast uncovered for 15 to 20 minutes, or until the chops register an internal temperature between 140° and 145°F.

4. To serve, remove the vegetables and fruit to a small mixing bowl and toss with the red wine vinegar. Spoon the mixture over the pork chops to serve. Garnish with fresh cilantro.

NIGHTSHADE-FREE

PORK LOIN WITH ROASTED RADISHES

I didn't learn to love radishes until I tried them roasted. Cooking at a high temperature mellows their peppery flavor and the chopped greens provide a beautiful contrast of color, flavor, and texture.

SERVES: 4 to 6   PREP TIME: 10 minutes   COOK TIME: 20 minutes

1 pound pork loin

3 tablespoons olive oil, divided

2 bunches radishes, thoroughly washed

juice of 1 lemon

sea salt

freshly ground pepper

1. Preheat the oven to 450°F. Line a sheet pan with parchment paper.

2. Pat the meat dry with paper towels. Coat with 1 tablespoon of the olive oil and season with salt and pepper. Place it on the center of the sheet pan.

3. Cut the tops off of the radishes and set the greens aside, leaving about 1 inch of the stem on each radish. Halve the radishes lengthwise and toss with the remaining 2 tablespoons of oil. Place them cut-side down on the sheet pan. Season with salt and pepper.

4. Roast uncovered for 20 minutes, or until the pork loin registers an internal temperature between 140° and 145°F.

5. Meanwhile, check the radish greens, removing any grit or wilted leaves, and then slice into thin ribbons.

6. Remove the pork to a cutting board and cover with foil for 10 minutes before slicing.

7. To serve, place the sliced pork in the center of a large serving platter and surround it with the roasted radishes. Top with the radish greens and shower with a big squeeze of lemon juice.

NIGHTSHADE-FREE ▪ LOW-FODMAP

ACORN SQUASH STUFFED WITH GROUND PORK, HAZELNUTS, AND SAGE

My birthday lands on the first day of autumn during some years, which predisposes me to love the season. Then again, what's not to love about the delicious flavors of fall? This recipe offers all of the savory ones in one dish.

SERVES: 4   PREP TIME: 10 minutes   COOK TIME: 40 to 45 minutes

2 acorn squash, halved

1 pound ground pork

1 small yellow onion, minced

1 celery stalk, minced

2 tablespoons minced fresh sage

1 teaspoon minced fresh thyme

½ teaspoon sea salt

¼ teaspoon freshly ground pepper

¼ cup roughly chopped toasted hazelnuts

1. Preheat the oven to 375°F. Line a sheet pan with parchment paper.

2. Cut the acorn squash in half and scoop out the seeds. Place the squash cut-side down on the sheet pan and roast for 20 minutes.

3. Meanwhile, combine the ground pork, onion, celery, herbs, salt, and pepper in a large bowl.

4. Remove the squash from the oven and turn cut-side up. Spoon the ground pork mixture into the squash loosely; do not pack it down. Sprinkle the top with the hazelnuts.

5. Return the pan to the oven and roast for another 15 to 20 minutes, or until the pork is browned and the squash is soft.

HOMEMADE ITALIAN SAUSAGE AND TOMATOES OVER ZUCCHINI NOODLES

Fennel seed and chile are the two spices that transform ordinary ground pork into the familiar flavors of Italian sausage. Want it spicier? Double the red chile flakes.

SERVES: 4   PREP TIME: 10 minutes   COOK TIME: 20 minutes

1 pound ground pork

1 yellow onion, minced

6 garlic cloves, divided

1 tablespoon fennel seed

½ teaspoon red chile flakes

1 pint grape tomatoes

2 tablespoons olive oil

1 cup roughly chopped fresh basil

2 zucchini

1. Preheat the oven to 375°F. Line a sheet pan with parchment paper.

2. Mince 2 of the garlic cloves and combine them with the ground pork, onion, fennel, and red chile flakes in a large bowl. Season with salt. Crumble the mixture onto half of the sheet pan.

3. Toss the grape tomatoes with the olive oil, basil, and remaining garlic cloves and spread onto the other half of the sheet pan. Season with salt

4. Roast uncovered for 20 to 25 minutes, until the pork is browned and the tomatoes are soft and bubbling.

5. Meanwhile, run the zucchini noodles through a spiralizer or use a vegetable peeler or mandoline to make long noodles. Divide the noodles among four bowls and top with the sausage and tomatoes.

BACON-LOADED BAKED POTATOES

Let's be honest—the best part of baked potatoes has always been the bacon (or maybe it's just me). If you choose to avoid potatoes, simply use small sweet potatoes in this recipe.

SERVES: 4   PREP TIME: 5 minutes   COOK TIME: 50 minutes

4 small russet potatoes, scrubbed and pierced with a fork

12 ounces applewood-smoked bacon

1 head broccoli, broken into very small florets

1 tablespoon olive oil

sea salt

freshly ground pepper

1. Preheat the oven to 400°F. Line a sheet pan with parchment paper.

2. As soon as the oven is preheated, place the potatoes directly onto the bottom rack of the oven.

3. Spread the broccoli on the sheet pan and toss with the olive oil. Season with salt and pepper.

4. Top the pan with an oven-safe baking rack and lay the bacon over the top.

5. Roast for 20 to 25 minutes, or until the bacon is crisp.

6. To serve, split the potatoes and crumble a few slices of bacon over each one and top with a generous heap of broccoli.

CITRUS AND HERB MARINATED PORK SHOULDER WITH SAVOY AND ALMOND SLAW

The long marinating time seasons this Cuban-style pork shoulder. Although a boneless piece of meat is much easier to slice, the bone-in pork stays nice and moist throughout the cooking process. Enjoy it over a simple cabbage and scallion slaw and top with almonds.

SERVES: 4 to 6   PREP TIME: 10 minutes, plus 8 to 12 hours for marinating   COOK TIME: 2 to 2½ hours

½ cup coconut oil

zest and juice of 3 to 4 oranges

zest and juice of 2 limes

1 cup plus 1 tablespoon fresh cilantro, divided

½ cup plus 1 tablespoon fresh mint leaves, divided

8 garlic cloves

2 teaspoons ground cumin

1 teaspoon ground coriander

3- to 4-pound bone-in pork shoulder

¼ cup olive oil

2 tablespoons lime juice

1 small head Savoy cabbage, thinly sliced

1 scallion, thinly sliced

½ cup toasted almond slices

sea salt

freshly ground pepper

1. In a large bowl, combine the coconut oil, citrus juices and zest, 1 cup of the cilantro, ½ cup of the mint, and the garlic, cumin, and coriander. Season with 1 teaspoon each of salt and pepper. Place the pork shoulder in the marinade and turn to coat thoroughly. Cover and refrigerate overnight.

2. Preheat the oven to 450°F. Place an oven-safe baking rack over a sheet pan.

3. Remove the pork shoulder from the marinade and set it on the rack. Season generously with salt and pepper. Roast uncovered for 30 minutes, then reduce the oven temperature to 325°F and cook for another 1½ to 2 hours, or until the pork is cooked to an internal temperature of 160°F.

4. Remove to a cutting board to rest for 15 to 20 minutes before slicing.

5. Mince the remaining cilantro and mint, and whisk it together with the olive oil and 2 tablespoons lime juice. Season with salt and pepper. Toss the cabbage, scallions, and almonds with the vinaigrette and serve alongside the sliced pork.

VIETNAMESE PORK MEATBALL LETTUCE WRAPS

I find deep satisfaction in creating dishes that I've eaten at a restaurant at home, and this one is hands-down one of my favorites. It replicates all of the delicious flavors you find in the Asian-fusion restaurants without the hefty price tag.

SERVES: 2 to 4   PREP TIME: 10 minutes   COOK TIME: 15 to 17 minutes

1 pound ground pork

1 tablespoon minced fresh ginger

1 teaspoon minced garlic

2 green onions, white and green parts, thinly sliced on a bias, divided

½ cup roughly chopped cilantro, divided

1 tablespoon fish sauce

1 cup shredded carrot

1 cup shredded cabbage

juice of 1 lime

leaves of 1 head butter lettuce

½ cup Cilantro Crema (page 253)

1. Preheat the oven to 400°F. Line a sheet pan with parchment paper.

2. Combine the pork, ginger, garlic, half of the green onions, half of the cilantro, and the fish sauce in a large bowl. Form into a dozen meatballs and place them on the sheet pan.

3. Bake uncovered for 10 minutes, then turn over and continue baking for another 5 to 7 minutes, or until the pork is cooked through.

4. While the meatballs are baking, combine the remaining green onion, cilantro, carrot, and cabbage. Squeeze the lime juice over the top.

5. To serve, place three meatballs in a lettuce leaf along with a heap of shredded carrot mixture and top with a drizzle of the cilantro crema.

CHAPTER SEVEN

Beef, Bison, & Veal

PEPPERCORN-CRUSTED BEEF SHORT RIBS WITH SORREL AND RADISHES

This is one of those dishes that you'll anticipate all week—partially because it takes nearly that long to prepare, but mostly because it's just so darn good! Don't worry, it's not all active prep time. The beef rests for 24 hours in the brine and another hour in the peppercorn crust. This is adapted from California-native chef Justin Smillie's recipe, as shared in Saveur magazine. My version cuts the prep and cooking time in half for a more succulent, juicy short rib. It also uses more easily accessible, Paleo-friendly ingredients.

SERVES: 2   PREP TIME: 45 minutes, plus 24 hours for brining
COOK TIME: 2 hours

1 cup plus 2 tablespoons assorted peppercorns (pink, green, white, and black), divided

1 tablespoon fennel seed

1 tablespoon coriander seed

½ cup plus 1 tablespoon coconut oil, divided

½ red onion, quartered

½ cup sea salt

2 tablespoons maple syrup

½ cup hot water

4 to 6 beef short ribs

large handful fresh sorrel leaves

small bunch radishes, thinly sliced

½ cup pitted kalamata olives

1 lemon, thinly sliced

2 tablespoons sherry vinegar

1. Heat 2 tablespoons of the peppercorns and the fennel and coriander seeds in a dry skillet over medium heat until gently toasted and aromatic, about 2 minutes. Pour them into a large glass dish.

2. Return the skillet to the heat and warm 1 tablespoon of the coconut oil. Cook the red onion pieces over medium-high heat until brown and caramelized, about 10 minutes. Add them to the glass dish.

3. Add the sea salt and maple syrup. Pour in the hot water. Stir to dissolve the salt. Add the short ribs. Pour in enough cool water to submerge the meat. Turn to coat the meat and disperse the flavors. Cover the dish and refrigerate for 24 hours (or up to 48).

4. Toast the remaining 1 cup of peppercorns over medium heat for 1 to 2 minutes. Add the remaining coconut oil. Simmer over low heat for 30 minutes. The aroma is breathtakingly floral. Allow the mixture to cool. Strain the peppercorns, allowing as much oil as possible to run off (save it for another use). Transfer them to a spice grinder or a mortar and pestle and pulverize until they resemble coarse sand.

5. Remove the short ribs from the brine. Pat dry with paper towels. Dredge the beef in the ground peppercorn mixture. Place them bone-side down on a sheet pan lined with parchment paper. Allow to rest at room temperature for up to an hour.

6. Preheat the oven to 375°F.

7. Cover the sheet pan tightly with foil. Roast for 1½ hours. Remove the foil and roast for another 30 minutes. The meat will be tender and falling off the bone. Allow to rest on the tray for 15 minutes before slicing the meat away from the bone and cutting into two pieces.

8. To serve, scatter the sorrel over a serving platter. Top with the meat, followed by the radishes, olives, and lemon slices. Drizzle with sherry vinegar.

KOREAN-STYLE SHORT RIBS WITH RED CABBAGE

The richness of the short ribs is perfectly offset by the tangy crunch of the cabbage in this easy weeknight supper. Simply toss the short ribs into the marinade in the morning and pull them out when you arrive home after a long workday. This recipe calls for flanken-cut short ribs, which is a method of cutting across the ribs instead of between them (English style). You'll likely need to request this cut specifically from your butcher.

SERVES: 2 to 4   PREP TIME: 10 minutes, plus up to 12 hours for marinating   COOK TIME: 12 minutes

2 tablespoons coconut aminos

2 tablespoons fish sauce

3 tablespoons rice wine vinegar, divided

2 teaspoons hot sauce

1 tablespoon coconut palm sugar

1 teaspoon sesame oil

2 garlic cloves, minced

1 teaspoon minced fresh ginger

1½ pounds flanken-cut beef short ribs, cut ½ inch thick and patted dry

4 to 6 cups shredded red cabbage

4 green onions, sliced paper thin on a bias

1. Combine the coconut aminos, fish sauce, 2 tablespoons of the rice wine vinegar, hot sauce, palm sugar, sesame oil, garlic, and ginger in a glass baking dish or bowl. Add the short ribs, cover, and marinate in the refrigerator for up to 12 hours.

2. Line a sheet pan with foil and top with an oven-safe baking rack. Remove the short ribs from the marinade, shaking off any excess. Place the ribs on top of the rack and allow to air-dry for about 30 minutes.

3. Preheat the broiler and place the oven rack on the top level, about 5 inches from the heating element. Broil the short ribs for 5 minutes, then flip over and broil for another 5 minutes. Remove the rack to a heat-safe countertop and pour the cabbage onto the pan, tossing to coat in any pan juices. Broil for 1 to 2 minutes, or until the cabbage is barely wilted. Season with the remaining 1 tablespoon rice wine vinegar and garnish with the green onions. Serve alongside the short ribs.

GROUND BEEF STUFFED BELL PEPPERS

If you're craving the flavors of tacos, these stuffed peppers are a Paleo-friendly nod to the Mexican mainstay. They're easy to make, and the filling can be prepared ahead of time to make weeknight meals a breeze.

SERVES: 2 to 4   PREP TIME: 15 minutes   COOK TIME: 30 minutes

4 sweet bell peppers, red, orange, and yellow

1 tablespoon coconut oil

1 yellow onion, diced

½ pound ground beef

2 garlic cloves, minced

1 tablespoon ground cumin

1 teaspoon smoked paprika

1 tablespoon tomato paste

¼ cup roughly chopped fresh cilantro

prepared guacamole, for serving

Pico de Gallo (page 250), for serving

1. Preheat the oven to 375°F. Line a sheet pan with parchment paper.

2. Remove the tops from the bell peppers with a paring knife.

3. Heat the coconut oil in a large skillet over medium heat. Cook the onion for 5 minutes, until slightly softened. Increase the heat to medium-high, add the ground beef, and cook until just browned.

4. Add the garlic and cook for another minute. Add the spices and tomato paste, and cook for 1 final minute. Remove from the heat and stir in the cilantro. Divide the mixture between the peppers.

5. Bake uncovered for 30 minutes. Serve with guacamole and pico de gallo.

STEAK AND BALSAMIC ASPARAGUS

It doesn't get any simpler than this—just five ingredients plus salt and pepper are all you need to get dinner on the table in a flash.

SERVES: 2 to 4   PREP TIME: 5 minutes   COOK TIME: 10 to 15 minutes

4 (6-ounce) New York Strip steaks, about 1 inch thick

1 bunch asparagus, trimmed

2 tablespoons olive oil, divided

2 tablespoons balsamic vinegar

1 teaspoon ground cumin

sea salt

freshly ground pepper

1. Preheat the oven to 350°F.

2. Toss the asparagus in 1 tablespoon of the oil and season generously with salt and pepper. Roast uncovered for 10 minutes on a sheet pan.

3. Meanwhile, heat the remaining 1 tablespoon oil in a large skillet until very hot. Season the steaks on both sides with salt and pepper. Brown for 2 to 3 minutes on each side.

4. Remove the pan from the oven and toss the asparagus with the balsamic vinegar and cumin. Make space between the asparagus spears and add the steaks.

5. Cook for another 5 to 10 minutes, or until the meat is cooked to your preference.

NIGHTSHADE-FREE · LOW-FODMAP

COWBOY MEATBALLS AND ONIONS

One evening I had a craving for beef and barbecue sauce and came up with this awesome Paleo meatball cooked with onions. If you include rice in your diet, it is delicious with the meatballs. You could also serve them with Sweet Potato Oven Fries (page 18).

SERVES: 4   PREP TIME: 5 minutes   COOK TIME: 20 minutes

2 yellow onions, halved then thinly sliced

2 tablespoons olive oil

1 teaspoon sea salt, divided

1 pound ground beef

2 tablespoons flax meal

½ cup minced onion

2 teaspoons smoked paprika

¼ cup minced uncooked bacon

2 eggs, whisked

1 cup Barbecue Sauce (page 245) or quality store-bought Paleo-friendly sauce

1. Preheat the oven to 375°F. Line a sheet pan with parchment paper.

2. Toss the onions with the olive oil and ½ teaspoon of the sea salt. Spread them out on the sheet pan and roast for 15 minutes.

3. Meanwhile, mix together the remaining ingredients, except the barbecue sauce, in a mixing bowl and form into 12 to 16 meatballs.

4. Remove the onions from the oven and stir. Add the meatballs and return the pan to the oven for another 15 minutes.

5. Pour the barbecue sauce over the meatballs and return to the oven for another 5 minutes, until the barbecue sauce is bubbling.

ITALIAN MEATBALLS WITH SPAGHETTI SQUASH

If you're a fan of spaghetti and meatballs but not so keen on cleaning a bunch of pots and pans, this dish is for you! The meatballs and spaghetti squash cook together, making cleanup a breeze.

SERVES: 4   PREP TIME: 5 minutes   COOK TIME: 40 minutes

1 spaghetti squash, about 1½ pounds sliced into 1-inch-thick rings, seeds removed

½ pound ground beef

½ pound ground pork

½ cup minced onion

2 tablespoons flax meal

½ teaspoon sea salt

1 teaspoon dried oregano

2 eggs, whisked

2 cups Roasted Tomato Marinara Sauce (page 244) or store-bought Paleo-friendly sauce

1 cup roughly chopped fresh basil

1. Preheat the oven to 400°F. Line a sheet pan with parchment paper.

2. Place the spaghetti squash rings on the sheet pan and roast uncovered for 20 minutes.

3. Meanwhile, mix together the remaining ingredients, except the marinara sauce and basil, in a large bowl and form into 8 large meatballs.

4. Place two meatballs in the center of each spaghetti squash ring. Roast for 15 minutes.

5. Pour the marinara sauce over the meatballs and return to the oven for another 5 minutes.

6. To serve, shred two spaghetti squash rings onto each plate and top with two meatballs and ¼ cup of basil.

BEEF TENDERLOIN AND PEPPER FAJITAS

This is a perfect dish to prepare all of the ingredients ahead of time and simply pop in the oven just before dinner. I'm always grateful for easy meals like this one after long days surfing, when the last thing I want to do is prepare a meal.

SERVES: 4 to 6   PREP TIME: 10 minutes   COOK TIME: 40 minutes

1 tablespoon smoked paprika

1 tablespoon ground cumin

1 teaspoon ground coriander

1¼ teaspoons sea salt, divided

3 tablespoons olive oil, divided

3 pound center-cut beef tenderloin

3 bell peppers, assorted colors, cut into 1-inch slices

2 yellow onions, halved then sliced in half circles

freshly ground pepper

leaves of 1 head butter lettuce

1 avocado, thinly sliced

½ cup roughly chopped fresh cilantro

1. Preheat the oven to 400°F. Line a sheet pan with parchment paper.

2. Combine the paprika, cumin, coriander, and 1 teaspoon of the salt in a small bowl. Pat the beef tenderloin dry with paper towels and then coat with 1 tablespoon of the olive oil. Press the spice rub into the meat. If you prepare it ahead of time, you can simply set it uncovered in the refrigerator.

3. Spread the peppers and onions on the sheet pan and toss with the remaining 2 tablespoons olive oil and ¼ teaspoon sea salt.

4. Set an oven-safe baking rack over the sheet pan and place the beef tenderloin in the center. Roast for 40 minutes or until the tenderloin reaches an internal temperature of 135° to 140°F. Allow the meat to rest for 10 minutes before slicing.

5. To serve, fill butter lettuce leaves with a few slices of beef and a spoonful of peppers and onions, and top with avocado and fresh cilantro.

COFFEE-CRUSTED BEEF TENDERLOIN WITH PARSNIPS

The crunch of the ground coffee is a pleasant textural contrast to the succulent beef tenderloin. The flavors are so lovely, I've paired them with a simple backdrop of roasted parsnips.

SERVES: 4 to 6   PREP TIME: 10 minutes   COOK TIME: 40 minutes

2 tablespoons ground coffee

2 tablespoons coconut palm sugar

1 tablespoon minced fresh rosemary

1¼ teaspoons sea salt, divided

1 teaspoon garlic powder

1 teaspoon onion powder

½ teaspoon red chile flakes

2 tablespoons olive oil, divided

3 pound center-cut beef tenderloin

4 to 6 parsnips, peeled and cut into 1-inch chunks

freshly ground pepper

1. Preheat the oven to 400°F. Line a sheet pan with parchment paper.

2. Combine the coffee, palm sugar, rosemary, 1 teaspoon of the sea salt, and the spices in a small bowl. Pat the beef tenderloin dry with paper towels and then coat with 1 tablespoon of the olive oil. Press the coffee rub into the meat. If you have extra time, wrap it in plastic wrap and set in the refrigerator for several hours to allow the flavors to permeate the meat.

3. Spread the parsnips on the sheet pan and toss with the remaining 1 tablespoon olive oil and ¼ teaspoon sea salt.

4. Set an oven-safe baking rack over the sheet pan and place the beef tenderloin in the center. Roast for 40 minutes, or until the tenderloin reaches an internal temperature of 135° to 140°F. Allow the meat to rest for 10 minutes before slicing and serving.

BEEF TENDERLOIN ROAST WITH STEWED VEGETABLES

There's something about tender beef roast paired with soft carrots, onions, and turnips that reminds me of my childhood. My mom used to make this dish in a crock-pot, but I find it works equally well in the oven, which allows the beef to maintain a lovely crust while the vegetables are melt-in-your-mouth tender.

SERVES: 4 to 6   PREP TIME: 10 minutes   COOK TIME: 50 to 60 minutes

- 3 pound center-cut beef tenderloin
- 1 tablespoons olive oil
- 1¼ teaspoons sea salt, divided
- 2 to 4 carrots with 1-inch of green tops, unpeeled and halved lengthwise
- 1 yellow onion, cut into 1-inch chunks
- 2 turnips, peeled and cut into 1-inch chunks
- 1 teaspoon minced fresh rosemary
- 1 teaspoon minced fresh thyme
- 1 cup dry red wine
- freshly ground pepper

1. Preheat the oven to 400°F.

2. Pat the beef tenderloin dry with paper towels and then coat with the olive oil. Season with 1 teaspoon of the salt and pepper.

3. Spread the carrots, onions, turnips, and herbs on the sheet pan and season with the remaining ¼ teaspoon of salt and pepper. Set the tenderloin in the center of the pan. Pour in the red wine.

4. Roast for 50 minutes to 1 hour or until the tenderloin reaches an internal temperature of 135° to 145°F. Allow the meat to rest for 10 minutes before slicing and serving.

NIGHTSHADE-FREE

FENNEL AND CHILE RUBBED RIBEYE STEAK WITH ROASTED RED PEPPERS

This spice rub will quickly become your new favorite for everything from beef and pork to chicken and even fish. Enjoy the steaks with a simple salad of mixed greens tossed in lemon juice.

SERVES: 4   PREP TIME: 10 minutes   COOK TIME: 15 minutes

¼ cup fennel seeds

2 tablespoons red chile flakes

1 tablespoon peppercorns

1 teaspoon sea salt

2 tablespoons coconut oil, divided

2 large ribeye steaks, at least 1 inch thick

2 red bell peppers, halved

8 cups mixed baby greens

juice of 1 lemon

1. Combine the fennel seeds, red chile flakes, and peppercorns in a spice grinder and blend until coarsely ground. Add the salt and pulse a few more times.

2. Pat the steaks dry with paper towels and rub with 1 tablespoon of the coconut oil. Press the spice rub into the steak. Allow to rest for 10 minutes or wrap in plastic and place in the refrigerator for up to 24 hours.

3. Preheat the broiler to high and place the oven rack about 8 inches from the heating element; the food should be about 5 inches from the element.

4. Coat the bell peppers in the remaining 1 tablespoon coconut oil. Place them on the sheet pan along with the ribeye steaks. Broil for 8 to 10 minutes, or until the peppers are charred. Remove them to a covered container to steam. Flip the steaks. Broil for another 5 to 10 minutes, or until the steak is cooked to an internal temperature of 135° to 140°F.

5. Allow the steaks to rest for 10 minutes before slicing. While they rest, remove the peppers, peel away the charred skin, and slice into long strips.

6. Toss the mixed greens with the lemon juice and serve alongside the steak and red peppers.

LOW-FODMAP

BEEF AND BROCCOLI TAKEOUT

This recipe is inspired by the classic Asian restaurant menu staple. Cooked without industrial oils, MSG, or heavy amounts of salt, it has a clean flavor you'll crave again and again.

SERVES: 2 to 4   PREP TIME: 10 minutes   COOK TIME: 20 minutes

1 head broccoli, cut into small florets

2 tablespoons olive oil, divided

1 tablespoon minced garlic

½ teaspoon red chile flakes

1 tablespoon coconut aminos

1 boneless ribeye steak, 1 to 1½ pounds

sea salt

freshly ground pepper

juice of 1 lime

1. Preheat the oven to 450°F. Line a sheet pan with parchment paper.

2. Spread the broccoli out on the sheet pan and toss with 1 tablespoon of the olive oil, garlic, red chile flakes, and coconut aminos.

3. Top the pan with an oven-safe baking rack. Season the steak with the remaining 1 tablespoon olive oil and season with salt and pepper. Set it atop the rack.

4. Roast for 10 minutes, then lower the temperature to 325°F and cook until the steak reaches an internal temperature of 135° to 140°F.

5. Allow the meat to rest for 10 minutes before slicing into very thin slices. Toss with the broccoli and season with the lime juice.

SLOW-ROASTED BARBECUE BEEF SHORT RIBS WITH ONIONS AND CARROTS

Short ribs are my new favorite cut of beef. The immense amount of fat is just delicious as it renders and keeps the meat juicy and tender. Seriously, so good!

SERVES: 4   PREP TIME: 5 minutes   COOK TIME: 3½ hours

3 to 4 pounds boneless beef short ribs, cut into 3-inch-long pieces

1 yellow onion, halved, then cut into thick half circles

1½ cups Barbecue Sauce (page 245) or store-bought Paleo-friendly barbecue sauce

6 to 8 small carrots, with 1-inch tops, halved lengthwise

1 tablespoon olive oil

sea salt

freshly ground pepper

1. Preheat the oven to 300°F.

2. Spread the short ribs and onions out on the sheet pan and season with sea salt and pepper. Drizzle the barbecue sauce over the top. Cover the sheet pan tightly with foil and bake for 2½ hours.

3. Coat the carrots in the olive oil.

4. Remove the foil from the sheet pan and add the carrots. Roast uncovered for another 30 minutes or until the meat is very tender and the carrots are cooked through

TRADITIONAL BRITISH PASTIES

So many cultures around the world have figured out this eternal truth: There's something incredibly comforting about pastry filled with meat. This Paleo version uses an almond flour pastry crust, which gets beautifully crispy but won't leave you with a grain hangover. Make sure to dice the meat and vegetables in the same size pieces so they cook evenly. Aim for about ¼ to ⅓ inch cubes.

SERVES: 4 to 6   PREP TIME: 20 minutes   COOK TIME: 40 to 45 minutes

4 cups blanched almond flour

2 tablespoons tapioca flour

1½ teaspoons sea salt, divided

5 tablespoons ice water

¼ cup palm shortening

1 large egg

½ pound beef skirt steak, cut into ⅓-inch dice

1 cup diced yellow or white onion

1 cup peeled, diced red or Yukon gold potatoes

1 cup diced carrots

freshly ground pepper

2 tablespoons olive oil

1 teaspoon chopped fresh thyme

1 teaspoon chopped fresh rosemary

1. Combine the almond flour, tapioca flour, and 1 teaspoon of the sea salt in a food processor and pulse once or twice. Add the ice water, palm shortening, and egg, and blend until thoroughly combined. Divide the mixture into 4 to 6 small balls (depending on how many pies you want) and place in the refrigerator.

2. Combine the steak, onion, potatoes, carrots, salt, pepper, olive oil, and herbs in a medium bowl.

3. Preheat the oven to 400°F. Line a sheet pan with parchment paper.

4. Remove the pastry from the refrigerator and roll a ball of dough between two sheets of parchment until it is a thin circle, about ⅛ inch thick. Remove the top square of parchment.

5. Place some of the meat and vegetable filling on the center of the pastry circle, slightly to one side. Pick up the parchment paper to fold the other side over and press the seam together. Carefully transfer the pie to the sheet pan. Repeat with the remaining pastry dough.

6. Bake uncovered for 40 to 45 minutes or until the crust is golden brown. Allow to rest for 10 minutes before serving.

BROILED FILET MIGNON WITH CHARRED LEEKS

Leeks are much more popular in France than they are in America, but we're slowly catching on to how awesome they are. These delicious vegetables have a more delicate flavor and texture than onions. Keep an eye on them during the final 5 minutes of cooking to make sure they don't burn. If they look like they might become overcooked, simply remove them to a warm platter while the steaks finish cooking. For a truly French experience, serve with Paleo Béarnaise Sauce (page 257).

SERVES: 4   PREP TIME: 10 minutes   COOK TIME: 25 minutes

4 leeks, white and pale green parts only, halved lengthwise

½ cup dry white wine

1 teaspoon fresh thyme

4 (½-pound) filet mignon steaks

2 tablespoons olive oil, divided

sea salt

freshly ground pepper

1. Preheat the oven to 400°F. Remove the steaks from the refrigerator to bring to room temperature.

2. Cut a large square of foil, set in onto a sheet pan, and place the leeks in it with the white wine and thyme. Season generously with salt and pepper. Fold into a tight pouch. Bake for 15 minutes.

3. Remove the pan from the oven, remove the leeks from the foil, and spread onto the sheet pan, cut-side up. Brush with 1 tablespoon of the olive oil.

4. Preheat the oven to broil. Set an oven-safe baking rack over the leeks on the sheet pan. Pat the steaks dry with paper towels and place them on the rack. Coat them with the remaining 1 tablespoon olive oil and season with salt and pepper.

5. Broil for 5 minutes, then flip the steaks and broil for another 5 minutes for medium rare. Allow the meat to rest for 10 minutes before plating and serving with the leeks.

NIGHTSHADE-FREE

LONDON BROIL WITH ROASTED SWEDE

London broil has no known origins in London. Nevertheless, it's pretty delicious with the classic English vegetable swede. I enjoyed it for the first time at a dimly lit restaurant in a little village on the border of England and Wales. At first I couldn't pinpoint what it even was and had to ask the server. In America, it's called a rutabaga or yellow turnip.

SERVES: 6 PREP TIME: 10 minutes, plus 4 to 6 hours for marinating
COOK TIME: 50 minutes

¼ cup red wine vinegar

½ cup hot water

1 tablespoon coconut palm sugar

1 tablespoon sea salt

1 sprig rosemary, needles only

1 tablespoon black peppercorns

1 cup ice water

3 pound flank steak

2 swedes (rutabagas), peeled and diced

3 tablespoons olive oil, divided

sea salt

freshly ground black pepper

1. Combine the vinegar, hot water, palm sugar, salt, rosemary, and peppercorns in a shallow dish. Stir until the sugar and salt are dissolved. Add the ice water. Add the flank steak, cover, and marinate for 4 to 6 hours in the refrigerator.

2. Preheat the oven to 400°F.

3. Toss the swedes with 2 tablespoons of the olive oil and season with salt and pepper. Place atop a large square of parchment paper, wrap into a tight package, and place on the sheet pan. Roast for 40 minutes.

4. Remove the pan from the oven and preheat the broiler. Place the oven rack on the top level, about 5 inches from the heating element.

Unfold the parchment, spreading the swedes out onto the pan. Top with an oven-safe baking rack.

5. Remove the meat from the marinade and pat dry with paper towels. Rub with the remaining 1 tablespoon olive oil. Place the marinated meat on top of the rack and place under the broiler for 5 minutes, then turn to the other side and broil for another 5 minutes, or until it reaches your desired level of doneness. Allow the meat to rest for 10 minutes before slicing and serving with the swedes.

NIGHTSHADE-FREE

LONDON BROIL OVER MIXED GREENS WITH BALSAMIC VINAIGRETTE

Enjoy this simple, elegant salad for lunch or a light dinner. I've included dates and apples here, because that's how I like it, but if you're watching carbs, feel free to omit them.

SERVES: 6   PREP TIME: 10 minutes, plus 4 hours for marinating   COOK TIME: 10 minutes

½ cup balsamic vinegar, divided

½ cup hot water

1 tablespoon coconut palm sugar

1 tablespoon sea salt

1 tablespoon black peppercorns

1 cup ice water

3 pound flank steak

4 tablespoons olive oil, divided

1 tablespoon minced shallots

1 teaspoon fresh thyme leaves

8 to 12 cups mixed greens such as frisee, baby romaine, and herbs

8 medjool dates, pitted and roughly chopped

2 apples, such as Pink Lady, julienned

sea salt

freshly ground black pepper

1. Combine ¼ cup of the vinegar, hot water, palm sugar, salt, and peppercorns in a shallow dish. Stir until the sugar and salt are dissolved. Add the ice water. Add the flank steak, cover, and marinate for 4 hours in the refrigerator.

2. Preheat the broiler and position the oven rack about 5 inches from the heating element.

3. Remove the meat from the marinade and pat dry with paper towels. Rub with 1 tablespoon of the olive oil. Place under the broiler for 5 minutes, then turn to the other side and broil for another 5 minutes, or until it reaches your desired level of doneness. Allow the meat to rest for 10 minutes before slicing.

4. While the steak is cooking, whisk together the remaining ¼ cup balsamic vinegar, 3 tablespoons olive oil, shallots, and thyme. Season to taste with salt and pepper.

5. Divide the greens among the plates and top with steak slices. Pour the vinaigrette over each salad and top with dates and apples.

NIGHTSHADE-FREE

GINGER AND GARLIC MARINATED FLANK STEAK LETTUCE WRAPS

Asian takeout is my go-to, and this ginger and garlic marinated flank steak re-creates some of my favorite flavors. If you can get your hands on some lemongrass, add one spear, split open and gently crushed, to the marinade.

SERVES: 2 to 4   PREP TIME: 10 minutes, plus 2 to 4 hours for marinating
COOK TIME: 10 minutes

¼ cup rice wine vinegar, divided

½ cup hot water

1 tablespoon coconut palm sugar

1 tablespoon sea salt

1 teaspoon red chile flakes

1 tablespoon minced fresh ginger

1 tablespoon minced garlic

1 spear lemongrass (optional)

1 cup ice water

1½ pounds flank steak

1 tablespoon toasted sesame oil

leaves of 1 to 2 heads butter lettuce

2 limes, cut into wedges, for serving

1 cup julienned carrots

½ cup fresh cilantro, for serving

sea salt

freshly ground black pepper

1. Combine ¼ cup of the vinegar, hot water, palm sugar, salt, chile flakes, ginger, garlic, and lemongrass, if using, in a shallow dish. Stir until the sugar and salt are dissolved. Add the ice water. Add the flank steak, cover, and marinate for 2 to 4 hours in the refrigerator.

2. Preheat the broiler and position the oven rack to about 5 inches from the heating element.

3. Remove the meat from the marinade and pat dry with paper towels. Rub with the sesame oil. Place under the broiler for 5 minutes, then turn to the other side and broil for another 5 minutes, or until it reaches your desired level of doneness. Allow the meat to rest for 10 minutes before slicing.

4. To serve, fill each lettuce leaf with a few slices of meat. Squeeze lime juice over it and top with carrots and cilantro.

BEEF RIB ROAST WITH NEW POTATOES

This is one of those special-occasion dishes that you should enjoy no matter the occasion. It has all of the seriousness of a gourmet meal but so much comfort, it will brighten even the darkest winter evening. To make it extra special, serve it with Classic French Red Wine Demi-Glace (page 258).

SERVES: 4   PREP TIME: 10 minutes   COOK TIME: 50 to 60 minutes

2 teaspoons minced garlic

2 teaspoons minced shallot

4 tablespoons olive oil, divided

3 pound beef rib roast with bones

1 pound new potatoes, cut into 1-inch cubes

1 teaspoon fresh rosemary

sea salt

freshly ground pepper

1. Preheat the oven to 350°F. Line a sheet pan with parchment paper.

2. Combine the garlic, shallots, and 2 tablespoons of the olive oil in a small dish. Spread it over the beef rib roast to coat and season with salt and pepper. Place the roast on the center of the pan.

3. Toss the potatoes with the rosemary and remaining 2 tablespoons olive oil. Season with salt and pepper. Scatter them around the roast.

4. Cook for 50 to 60 minutes, or until the roast reaches an internal temperature of 120°F.

SIMPLE PRIME RIB ROAST WITH VEGETABLES

This prime rib roast is simplicity at its finest. Just a little thinking ahead will give it loads of flavor.

SERVES: 4 to 6   PREP TIME: 15 minutes, plus 8 to 12 hours resting time
COOK TIME: 1½ to 2 hours

1 head garlic

1 sprig rosemary

1 (3- to 4-pound) center-cut prime rib roast

4 tablespoons rendered bacon fat, divided

4 carrots, cut into 2-inch pieces

4 potatoes, quartered

2 yellow onions, quartered

1 tablespoon fresh thyme

sea salt

freshly ground black pepper

1. Peel the garlic cloves and remove the needles from the rosemary sprig. Make several slits in the prime rib. Stuff a clove and rosemary needle into each hole. Cover and refrigerate overnight.

2. Remove the meat from the refrigerator at least an hour before placing in the oven to allow it to come to room temperature.

3. Preheat the oven to 450°F. Coat the meat in 2 tablespoons of the bacon fat and season liberally with salt and pepper. Roast uncovered for 30 minutes to brown. Remove the pan from the oven. Reduce the heat to 325°F and bake for another 30 minutes

4. Toss the carrots, potatoes, onions, and thyme with the remaining bacon fat and season with salt and pepper. Spread the vegetables around the roast and return the pan to the oven. Roast for another hour, or until the roast reaches an internal temperature of 140°F. Remove to a cutting board and allow to rest for 20 minutes before serving with the vegetables.

ROASTED BEEF MARROW BONES WITH LEMON ASPARAGUS

If you haven't yet tried it, roasted bone marrow will be a pleasant and flavorful surprise. Ask your butcher to cut the marrow bones for you.

SERVES: 2   PREP TIME: 5 minutes   COOK TIME: 15 minutes

4 (3-inch) pieces beef marrow bones

1 bunch asparagus, trimmed

1 tablespoon olive oil

zest and juice of 1 lemon

sea salt

freshly ground pepper

1. Preheat the oven to 425°F. Line a sheet pan with parchment paper.

2. Place the marrow bones on the pan, cut-side up.

3. Toss the asparagus with the olive oil and lemon zest and spread around the bones. Season the whole pan with salt and pepper.

4. Roast uncovered for 15 minutes or until the marrow is bubbling.

5. Drizzle the asparagus with the lemon juice just before serving.

NIGHTSHADE-FREE

OSSO BUCO

I first encountered osso buco while working at an Italian restaurant in downtown Portland, Oregon, where we served it with a small table knife stuck into the marrow. It was clearly a delicacy, but I had no idea how healthy bone marrow is and how prized it has been for millennia for its nutrient density and creamy, rich flavor.

SERVES: 4   PREP TIME: 15 minutes   COOK TIME: 2 hours and 5 minutes

4 pieces veal shank

2 tablespoons olive oil

1 onion, halved then sliced in thin half circles

1 celery stalk, diced

1 carrot, diced

4 garlic cloves, minced

1 teaspoon fresh rosemary

1 teaspoon fresh thyme

2 bay leaves

2 cinnamon sticks

1 (15-ounce) can plum tomatoes, drained

2 cups dry red wine

sea salt

freshly ground pepper

1. Preheat the broiler and position the oven rack to about 5 inches from the heating element.

2. Rub the veal shanks on all sides with olive oil and season with salt and pepper. Broil for 2 to 3 minutes, or until browned, then flip and brown on the other side. Remove the pan from the oven and turn the oven temperature to bake at 375°F.

3. Add the remaining ingredients to the pan around the veal shanks, pouring in wine until it comes partially up the side of the sheet pan. Season with salt and pepper.

4. Cover the pan tightly with foil and bake for 1½ hours.

5. Remove the foil and bake for another 30 minutes. The meat will be falling off the bone and the vegetables very soft.

BISON BURGERS WITH BACON MAYO

The first time I made these savory burgers, I thought, it doesn't get any more Paleo than this. (Of course, that was before I tried Roast Turkey Legs with Brussels Sprouts, page 116.) Trust me on the bacon mayo— it's just exquisite.

SERVES: 4   PREP TIME: 5 minutes   COOK TIME: 15 to 20 minutes

1 pound ground bison

1 teaspoon minced garlic

1 shallot, minced

½ teaspoon sea salt, divided

¼ teaspoon freshly ground pepper

1 small yellow onion, thinly sliced

1 tablespoon olive oil

8 butter lettuce leaves

½ cup Bacon Mayo (page 252)

2 tomatoes, thinly sliced

1. Preheat the oven to 375°F. Line a sheet pan with parchment paper.

2. Mix together the bison, garlic, shallots, ¼ teaspoon of the salt, and pepper. Form into 4 patties, about 1 inch thick and place on the sheet pan.

3. Place the onion slices on the sheet pan and coat in the olive oil and remaining salt.

4. Roast uncovered for 15 to 20 minutes, or until the burgers are cooked through.

5. To serve, use the butter lettuce leaves as buns and top each burger with a generous dollop of Bacon Mayo and then top with the onions, tomatoes, and another lettuce leaf. Serve immediately.

NIGHTSHADE-FREE

BISON TRI-TIP ROAST WITH TURNIP, PARSNIP, AND SWEET POTATOES

Large cuts of meat do well with oven roasting because they have time to brown on the outside and remain succulent and moist on the inside. Bison often has a more tender texture than does beef, and the price reflects it.

SERVES: 4 PREP TIME: 10 minutes COOK TIME: 55 minutes

2½ pounds bison tri-tip roast, silver skin removed

4 tablespoons olive oil, divided

1 teaspoon minced fresh rosemary

1 teaspoon fresh thyme

1 large sweet potato, peeled and diced

3 to 4 parsnips, peeled and diced

1 turnip, peeled and diced

sea salt

freshly ground pepper

1. Preheat the oven to 450°F. Line a sheet pan with parchment paper.

2. Coat the bison in 2 tablespoons of the olive oil and season with the herbs, salt, and pepper. Allow to rest at room temperature while preparing the other ingredients or refrigerate for up to 8 hours.

3. Spread the sweet potatoes, parsnips, and turnips on the sheet pan and toss with the remaining 2 tablespoons olive oil and season with salt and pepper. Place the bison in the center of the pan, pushing the vegetables to the side to make room.

4. Roast uncovered for 15 minutes, then reduce the oven temperature to 325°F and cook for another 30 to 40 minutes, or until the bison reaches an internal temperature of 140°F. Remove the meat to a cutting board and allow it to rest for 15 minutes, where the internal temperature will continue to rise. Serve with the vegetables.

BISON BOURGUIGNON

Compared to beef, bison is quite lean, with a very fine marbling of fat. Braising it low and slow in red wine is one way to keep it tender and moist. You don't have to brown the meat before placing it on the sheet pan, but it will impart a beautiful, rich flavor to the dish. To save time, purchase frozen pearl onions, which have already been blanched and skinned. Simply defrost before placing them on the sheet pan.

SERVES: 4   PREP TIME: 15 minutes   COOK TIME: 2 to 2½ hours

2 tablespoons rendered bacon fat

2 to 3 pounds bison brisket, cut into 1-inch pieces

2 cups pearl onions, blanched and skinned

2 carrots, diced

2 cups mushrooms, halved

1 tablespoon fresh thyme leaves

2 to 3 cups red wine

sea salt

freshly ground pepper

1. Preheat the oven to 325°F.

2. Heat the bacon fat in a large skillet over medium-high heat. Season the bison with the salt and pepper and brown on all sides. You may have to do this in batches so as not to crowd the pan.

3. Place the browned meat onto a sheet pan. Add the onions, carrots, mushrooms, and thyme, and pour in the wine so it comes partially up the sides of the sheet pan.

4. Cover the pan tightly with aluminum foil. Roast for 1½ to 2 hours. Remove the foil and cook for another 30 minutes to reduce the liquid slightly and yield fork-tender meat.

NIGHTSHADE-FREE

VEAL MARSALA

I'm in love with the complex sweetness of Marsala. Make sure to purchase real Marsala wine, not the cooking wine sold next to vinegars.

SERVES: 4   PREP TIME: 10 minutes   COOK TIME: 25 to 35 minutes

2 large shallots, minced

2 garlic cloves, minced

8 ounces cremini mushrooms, thinly sliced

4 tablespoons olive oil, divided

1 pound veal cutlets

¼ cup potato starch

1 cup Marsala wine

sea salt

freshly ground pepper

1. Preheat the oven to 350°F.

2. Spread the shallots, garlic, and mushrooms out on the sheet pan. Drizzle with 2 tablespoons of the olive oil. Season with salt and pepper.

3. Heat the remaining 2 tablespoons olive oil over medium-high heat in a large skillet.

4. Season the veal cutlets with salt and pepper then dredge in the potato starch, shaking off any excess. Brown the cutlets in the skillet for 2 to 3 minutes on each side. Place on top of the mushrooms on the sheet pan. Pour the Marsala over the veal cutlets. Place in the oven and roast uncovered for 20 to 30 minutes. The veal will be tender and the mushrooms fragrant and browned.

VEAL SHOULDER WITH WILD MUSHROOMS AND RED WINE DEMI-GLACE

The flavors of veal, wild mushrooms, and rich red wine demi-glace meld beautifully in this ultimate comfort-food dish. The veal shoulder can be browned using the broiler if you prefer to only use the sheet pan and oven, but a stovetop method is more conventional and efficient.

SERVES: 6 to 8   PREP TIME: 10 minutes   COOK TIME: 2½ to 3 hours

1 ounce dried wild mushrooms

2 tablespoons minced garlic

1 teaspoon minced fresh rosemary

1 teaspoon minced fresh thyme

1 teaspoon sea salt

½ teaspoon freshly ground black pepper

1 (4- to 5-pound) veal shoulder roast

4 tablespoons olive oil, divided

1 cup diced celery

2 yellow onions, sliced in thick rings

4 carrots, cut into 2-inch pieces

1 cup Classic French Red Wine Demi-Glace (page 258)

1. Process the dried mushrooms in a spice grinder until finely ground. Mix them with the garlic, herbs, salt, and pepper. Spread the mixture on all sides of the veal shoulder and then roll into a cylinder and tie with kitchen twine.

2. Heat 2 tablespoons of the olive oil over medium-high heat in a large skillet. Brown the veal on all sides then place on the sheet pan.

3. Spread the celery, onions, and carrots on the pan around the veal. Drizzle with the remaining 2 tablespoons olive oil and season with salt and pepper. Spread the demi-glace over the meat and cover the pan tightly with foil. Bake for 2½ to 3 hours.

4. Allow the meat to rest for 15 minutes before slicing. Place it in the center of the sheet pan, surround with the vegetables, and drizzle with the pan juices.

BROILED VEAL CHOPS WITH SMASHED HERBED POTATOES

Simply marinate these veal chops ahead of time and then place them under the broiler for 10 minutes for a quick and satisfying dinner.

SERVES: 4   PREP TIME: 10 minutes, plus 3 hours for marinating
COOK TIME: 40 minutes

3 garlic cloves, minced

1 tablespoon herbes de Provence

½ cup white wine

¼ cup olive oil

zest and juice of 1 lemon

½ teaspoon sea salt

½ teaspoon freshly ground pepper

4 (12-ounce) veal chops

1 dozen Yukon gold potatoes

¼ cup chopped fresh parsley

1. Combine the garlic, herbes de Provence, wine, olive oil, lemon zest and juice, salt, and pepper in a small bowl. Spread it over the veal chops, reserving ¼ cup of the mixture for the potatoes. Allow the veal chops to rest in a covered container in the refrigerator for at least 3 hours, and up to 8 hours.

2. Preheat the oven to 350°F and line a sheet pan with parchment paper. Poke several holes in the potatoes and roast on the sheet pan for 30 minutes.

3. Remove the pan from the oven and smash each of the potatoes with the flat side of a meat cleaver or the back of a skillet. Drizzle the remaining herb marinade over the potatoes.

4. Preheat the broiler and place the oven rack about 5 inches from the element.

5. Top the potatoes with an oven-safe baking rack and place the veal chops on the rack. Broil for 5 minutes, then flip the chops and broil for another 5 minutes. Keep an eye on the potatoes. They should be protected from the direct heat of the element by the veal chops, but make sure they toast but do not burn.

6. Cut the veal in thin slices and serve with the smashed potatoes.

ROASTED RACK OF VEAL

Paleo entertaining doesn't get much more luxurious than a dramatic roasted rack of veal. Crisscross the racks on the sheet pan for an especially impressive presentation. If you're serving wine, go for a Pinot Noir. I grew up in Oregon, so I'm partial to those from the Willamette Valley.

SERVES: 8   PREP TIME: 10 minutes, plus 8 hours for marinating
COOK TIME: 1½ hours

¼ cup olive oil

3 tablespoons garlic, divided

2 tablespoons smoked paprika

2 tablespoons minced fresh sage

1 tablespoon plus 1 teaspoon minced fresh rosemary, divided

1 tablespoon plus 1 teaspoon fresh thyme leaves, divided

1 tablespoon sea salt

1 teaspoon freshly ground pepper

2 veal racks, 5 bones each, frenched

1 pound assorted mushrooms, larger ones halved

½ cup red wine

1. Combine the olive oil, 2 tablespoons of the garlic, paprika, sage, 1 tablespoon each of the rosemary and thyme, salt, and pepper in a small bowl and whisk into a thick paste. Spread this on the veal racks, cover with plastic wrap, and refrigerate for at least 8 hours and up to 24 hours. Allow the veal to come to room temperature before roasting.

2. Preheat the oven to 450°F. Line a sheet pan with parchment paper.

3. Place the veal racks on the center of the sheet pan with the bones crisscrossing one another. Roast for 15 minutes, then reduce the oven temperature to 350°F and roast for another hour.

4. During the last 30 minutes of cooking, toss the mushrooms with the remaining garlic and herbs, and pour in the wine. Season with salt and pepper. Spread the mixture out on the sheet pan.

5. When the veal racks have reached an internal temperature of 130°F, remove them to a cutting board and tent with foil for 15 minutes. They will continue cooking outside of the oven.

6. While the veal rests, allow the mushrooms to continue cooking until they are wilted and the wine has reduced. Serve alongside the veal.

CHAPTER EIGHT

Lamb & Goat

HERBED LAMB SHOULDER WITH SWEET POTATO FRIES

The grassy flavor of the herbs complements the slight gamey flavor of lamb. This dish is delicious with a Marlborough Sauvignon Blanc.

SERVES: 2   PREP TIME: 10 minutes, plus up to 24 hours for marinating
COOK TIME: 35 to 45 minutes

¼ cup plus 3 tablespoons olive oil, divided

2 tablespoons sherry vinegar or red wine vinegar

¼ cup minced fresh parsley

¼ cup minced fresh mint

1 shallot, minced (about ¼ cup)

2 garlic cloves, minced

3/4 teaspoon sea salt, divided

2 lamb shoulder chops, about 8 ounces each

1 large sweet potato, unpeeled

freshly ground pepper

1. In a medium bowl, combine ¼ cup of the olive oil with the vinegar, parsley, mint, shallots, garlic, ½ teaspoon of the salt, and several grinds of pepper. Use an immersion blender to puree to an almost smooth consistency.

2. Pour over the lamb shoulder chops and marinate while you prepare and roast the sweet potato, or up to 24 hours in the refrigerator.

3. Preheat the oven to 375°F.

4. Cut the sweet potato into ¼-inch spears. Coat in the remaining 3 tablespoons olive oil and place on a sheet pan, leaving space for the lamb chops. Sprinkle with the remaining ¼ teaspoon sea salt. Bake for 15 to 20 minutes.

5. Add the lamb chops to the pan. Bake for another 20 to 25 minutes until the lamb is cooked through to an internal temperature of 145°F.

NIGHTSHADE-FREE

MOROCCAN SPICE-RUBBED LEG OF LAMB

For the best flavor, toast the coriander and cumin seeds whole before grinding. Simply heat a dry skillet over medium heat and shake it gently to toast the spices evenly. Continue cooking until they're beautifully fragrant, about 2 to 3 minutes. Grind in a spice grinder or a mortar and pestle. Serve the finished dish with a small salad or white rice, if you choose to include it in your diet.

SERVES: 6   PREP TIME: 10 minutes   COOK TIME: 1½ hours

1 bone-in leg of lamb, about 6 pounds

¼ cup lime juice

1 tablespoon ground coriander

1 tablespoon ground cumin

1 tablespoon curry powder

2 tablespoons minced garlic

6 to 8 carrots, whole, peeled

1 yellow onion, sliced in ½-inch rings

1 tablespoon olive oil

sea salt

freshly ground pepper

1. Preheat the oven to 400°F.

2. Coat the lamb with the lime juice and then rub the spices and garlic into the meat. Season generously with salt and pepper.

3. Place the lamb on the sheet pan. Roast for 30 minutes uncovered, and then reduce the heat to 350°F and cook for another hour until the lamb is cooked through to an internal temperature of 145°F.

4. Toss the carrots and onion in the oil and add to the sheet pan for the last 45 minutes of cooking time. Allow the lamb to rest for 10 minutes before slicing and serving with the vegetables.

SLOW-ROASTED GARLIC AND THYME LEG OF LAMB WITH PARSNIPS

Cooking low and slow yields an even, tender piece of meat. In this recipe, it is cooked atop pieces of onion for flavor and aromatics.

SERVES: 6   PREP TIME: 10 minutes   COOK TIME: 3 hours

1 yellow onion, cut into ½-inch-thick slices

1 bone-in leg of lamb (about 6 pounds)

3 tablespoons olive oil, divided

2 tablespoons fresh thyme

2 tablespoons minced garlic

zest of 1 lemon

sea salt

4 parsnips, peeled

freshly ground pepper

1. Preheat the oven to 325°F. Line a sheet pan with parchment paper.

2. Scatter the onion slices across the sheet pan, breaking them up to separate the rings from one another. Toss with 1 tablespoon of the oil to coat.

3. Rub the lamb leg with 1 tablespoon of the oil and then coat with the thyme, garlic, and lemon zest. Season generously with salt and pepper.

4. Place the meat atop the onion slices. Bake uncovered for 2½ to 3 hours.

5. Cut the parsnips into ½-inch-thick spears. Toss with the remaining tablespoon of oil. Season generously with salt and pepper. In the final hour of cooking, place the parsnips atop the onion slices and return the pan to the oven.

6. Use an instant-read thermometer to gauge doneness on the meat: 125° to 130°F indicates medium rare, and 130° to 135°F indicates medium. Serve the lamb with the parsnips.

NIGHTSHADE-FREE

LAMB KEBABS WITH TAHINI, CUCUMBER, AND OLIVES

In college I worked at a Lebanese restaurant where I fell in love with Middle Eastern flavors. These lamb kebabs take me right back.

SERVES: 2 to 4   PREP TIME: 15 minutes   COOK TIME: 12 to 15 minutes

1 pound thick-cut boneless lamb chops, cut into 1-inch cubes

1 red bell pepper, cut into 1½-inch pieces

1 red onion, cut into 1½-inch pieces

¼ cup olive oil

1 teaspoon smoked paprika

1 teaspoon ground cumin

½ cup tahini

1 teaspoon minced garlic

juice of 1 lemon

1 English cucumber, sliced into spears

1 cup kalamata olives

sea salt

freshly ground pepper

1. Preheat the oven to 350°F. Line a sheet pan with parchment paper. Soak 6 bamboo or wooden skewers in water for at least 5 minutes.

2. Thread the meat, bell peppers, and onion onto the skewers. Coat them thoroughly in the olive oil and season with paprika, cumin, salt, and pepper. Lay the kebabs on the sheet pan.

3. Roast uncovered for 12 to 15 minutes, or until the meat is cooked to your desired level of doneness.

4. While the meat cooks, whisk together the tahini, garlic, and lemon juice. Serve the kebabs with the tahini sauce for dipping alongside the cucumber spears and kalamata olives.

SPICY SPANISH LAMB STEW

My husband traveled to Spain for a photography assignment and brought back a few bottles of vinegar and sherry for me. I'm always thrilled to try new flavors from around the globe and love the way they permanently influence my evolving cooking style. Serve this stew with Paleo-friendly almond flour flatbread or white rice. This dish calls for piment d'espelette, which is a chile cultivated in the Basque country located on the border between France and Spain. You can purchase the spice online or in a specialty market.

SERVES: 4   PREP TIME: 15 minutes, plus up to 8 hours for marinating
COOK TIME: 1½ to 2 hours

3 pounds lamb shoulder, cubed

1 tablespoon minced garlic

1 teaspoon minced fresh rosemary

2 teaspoons piment d'espelette or paprika

½ cup dry Spanish sherry

½ teaspoon sea salt

1 yellow onion, diced

2 roasted red bell peppers, sliced in thin pieces

½ cup fresh parsley, plus more for garnish

2 tablespoons olive oil

1½ cups Tempranillo or other full-bodied red wine

1. Combine the lamb, garlic, rosemary, piment d'espelette or paprika, and sherry in a nonreactive dish and toss to coat thoroughly. Cover and allow to marinate for at least 2 hours and up to 8 hours in the refrigerator.

2. Preheat the oven to 325°F.

3. Remove the lamb to the sheet pan and add the onions, red bell peppers, parsley, and olive oil. Pour in the wine until it comes partially up the sides of the pan. Cover the pan tightly with foil.

4. Bake for 1½ to 2 hours, and then remove the foil and roast uncovered for another 30 minutes until the meat is very tender.

EGGPLANT STUFFED WITH GROUND LAMB AND MEDITERRANEAN SPICES

I first enjoyed a version of this dish during a neighborhood potluck where I don't think I tried anything else. I just kept going back for helping after helping of pillowy eggplant and spiced lamb.

SERVES: 4   PREP TIME: 15 minutes   COOK TIME: 1½ hours

2 eggplants, sliced lengthwise

3 tablespoons olive oil, divided

1 yellow onion, minced

1 pound ground lamb

1½ teaspoons ground cumin

1 tablespoon smoked paprika

1 tablespoon ground cinnamon

1 tablespoon tomato paste

juice of ½ lemon

½ cup fresh parsley

sea salt

freshly ground pepper

1. Preheat the oven to 425°F.

2. Place the eggplants skin-side down on a sheet pan. Brush with 2 tablespoons of the olive oil and season generously with salt. Bake for 20 minutes.

3. Meanwhile, heat the remaining 1 tablespoon of olive oil in a wide skillet over medium heat. Add the onions and cook for about 10 minutes, until soft. Push it to the side. Increase the heat to medium-high. Place the ground lamb in the pan. Cook until just browned, about 5 to 7 minutes.

4. Add the spices and tomato paste, and stir to combine. Season with salt and pepper.

5. Spoon the lamb mixture over the eggplants. Carefully cover the pan with foil and bake for an hour. Remove the foil and continue cooking for about 15 minutes longer, until gently browned on the surface. Allow to rest for 10 minutes before serving. To serve, sprinkle the eggplants with lemon juice and minced fresh parsley.

CROWN ROAST OF LAMB WITH PARSNIP PUREE

It doesn't get much more impressive than a proud crown roast of lamb. Ask your butcher to french the racks for you, or watch a video online to learn how to do it yourself. Save this for special occasions and serve with a nice bottle of red wine.

SERVES: 4 to 6   PREP TIME: 10 minutes   COOK TIME: 50 minutes

2 racks lamb, frenched (about 2 pounds total)

4 tablespoons olive oil, divided

1 tablespoon fresh thyme leaves

1 tablespoon minced rosemary

1 teaspoon Dijon mustard

1 teaspoon sea salt

1 teaspoon freshly ground pepper

6 to 8 parsnips, peeled and cut into 1-inch pieces

1 tablespoon honey

½ cup coconut cream

1 cup chicken broth

1. Preheat the oven to 375°F. Line a sheet pan with parchment paper.

2. Bend each of the lamb racks into a half circle and tie with kitchen twine at the base and center. The rib ends should protrude from the top of the meat outward, like a crown.

3. Make a paste with 2 tablespoons of the olive oil, thyme, rosemary, mustard, salt, and pepper. Coat the racks of lamb with this mixture and set them on one side of the sheet pan.

4. Place the parsnips on a large square of foil. Drizzle with the remaining 2 tablespoons olive oil and season with salt and pepper. Fold the foil into a tight package and place on the sheet pan next to the lamb.

5. Roast for 35 minutes, or until the lamb reaches an internal temperature of 130°F. Remove the meat to a cutting board and tent with foil.

6. Allow the parsnips to continue baking for another 15 minutes. Open the package carefully and transfer the cooked parsnips to a blender. Add the honey, coconut cream, and chicken broth. Place a towel over the lid and then pulse a few times. Remove the lid to allow steam to escape, then puree until smooth. Serve the puree alongside the lamb.

FRENCH BRAISED LAMB SHANKS

Low, slow cooking is the key to perfect fall-off-the-bone lamb shanks. The vegetables melt into an almost sauce-like consistency.

SERVES: 4   PREP TIME: 10 minutes   COOK TIME: 1 hour 45 minutes

2 yellow onions, diced

2 celery stalks, diced

2 carrots, diced

1 leek, white and pale green parts only, sliced

4 plum tomatoes, quartered lengthwise

1 tablespoon herbes de Provence

2 tablespoons olive oil

4 (½- to ¾-pound) lamb shanks

½ cup Classic French Red Wine Demi-Glace (page 258)

sea salt

freshly ground pepper

1. Preheat the oven to 350°F.

2. Spread the onions, celery, carrot, leeks, tomatoes, and herbes de Provence out on a sheet pan. Toss with the olive oil and season with salt and pepper.

3. Nestle the lamb shanks in among the vegetables. Pour the demi-glace over the top of the meat and vegetables. Cover the pan tightly with foil.

4. Cook for 1 hour, then remove the foil and continue cooking for another 30 to 45 minutes, until the lamb reaches an internal temperature of 140° to 145°F and the meat has browned. Allow it to rest for 15 minutes before serving.

GOAT CURRY

Goat is the most widely consumed meat in the world, but many Americans are unfamiliar with its flavor and rarely see it in their local grocery stores. Fortunately, it is slowly edging its way into the mainstream market thanks in part to small farms and artisan restaurants. Because it has a decidedly gamey flavor, it does well with heavily spiced dishes such as this Indian curry. Feel free to use a Dutch oven or glass baking dish to easily contain the liquid in this stew.

SERVES: 4 PREP TIME: 10 minutes, plus 2 hours for marinating COOK TIME: 2 to 3 hours

2 pounds boneless goat leg meat, cut into 1-inch pieces

juice of 1 lemon

1 tablespoon minced fresh ginger

1 tablespoon minced garlic

3 tablespoons curry powder

½ teaspoon red chile flakes

1 teaspoon garam masala

1 yellow onion, diced

2 tomatoes, diced

¼ cup golden raisins

1 (15-ounce) can coconut milk

1 cup water, or as needed

½ cup fresh cilantro, for garnish

sea salt

freshly ground pepper

1. Combine the goat meat with the lemon juice, ginger, garlic, curry powder, red chile flakes, and garam masala. Season with salt and pepper. Cover and allow to rest in the refrigerator for 2 hours.

2. Preheat the oven to 325°F.

3. Spread the goat meat out on a sheet pan and toss with the onion, tomatoes, and raisins. Pour the coconut milk over the top and toss gently to combine. Pour in enough water to come partially up the sides of the sheet pan.

4. Cover the pan tightly with foil and roast for 2 to 3 hours, or until the meat is tender. Sprinkle with cilantro to serve.

ROSEMARY-GARLIC GOAT CHOPS

Pungent garlic and rosemary are a classic match for goat chops. Allow them to sit in the marinade for a few hours to deepen the flavor. Serve with simple cucumber spears and a side salad with a squeeze of lemon and drizzle of olive oil.

SERVES: 2 to 4   PREP TIME: 10 minutes, plus 3 hours for marinating   COOK TIME: 10 minutes

3 garlic cloves, minced

2 teaspoons minced fresh rosemary

2 tablespoons olive oil

4 goat rib chops

sea salt

freshly ground pepper

1. Combine the garlic, rosemary, and olive oil in a small bowl, and season with salt and pepper. Spread the mixture onto the goat chops. Cover and allow to rest in the refrigerator for 2½ hours. Remove 30 minutes before cooking to allow them to come to room temperature.

2. Preheat the broiler. Line a sheet pan with foil. Place an oven rack in the top position so the meat will be about 5 inches from the heating element.

3. Broil the ribs for 3 minutes, then flip and broil on the other side. Allow the meat to rest for 5 minutes before serving.

NIGHTSHADE-FREE

CHAPTER NINE

Game & Offal

BROILED QUAIL WITH ZUCCHINI AND PEACHES

Enjoy the flavors of summer in this delicious broiled quail dish. Bonus: With just 10 minutes under the broiler, the meal won't heat up your kitchen!

SERVES: 4   PREP TIME: 10 minutes   COOK TIME: 10 minutes

6 whole jumbo quail (6 to 8 ounces each)

1 tablespoon minced fresh ginger

1 teaspoon minced garlic

2 tablespoons red wine vinegar

4 tablespoons olive oil, divided

4 ripe peaches, quartered

2 zucchini, cut into 1-inch pieces

1 teaspoon minced fresh rosemary

sea salt

freshly ground pepper

1. Using kitchen shears, cut the quail in half lengthwise, reserving the necks, feet, and first 2 wing joints for another use.

2. Combine the ginger, garlic, vinegar, 3 tablespoons of the olive oil, a pinch of salt, and a few grinds of pepper in a glass bowl. Add the quail halves and toss to coat thoroughly. You can do this step in advance and allow the quail to sit in the marinade in a covered container for up to 4 hours in the refrigerator.

3. Toss the peaches and zucchini in the remaining 1 tablespoon oil and season with the rosemary, salt, and pepper.

4. Preheat the broiler and place a rack on the top of the oven, about 5 inches from the heating element. Line a sheet pan with parchment paper. Spread the quail, zucchini, and peaches out on the sheet pan.

5. Broil for 5 minutes, then turn the quail over and broil for another 3 to 5 minutes, until the quail is cooked through and the juices run clear.

NIGHTSHADE-FREE

BACON-WRAPPED QUAIL WITH DICED SWEET POTATOES

My friend Natalie grew up enjoying bacon-wrapped quail stuffed with jalapeño and encouraged me to include the recipe here. The flavors are like a punch in the face—in a good way!

SERVES: 4   PREP TIME: 10 minutes   COOK TIME: 15 to 20 minutes

- 8 small whole quail (about 4 ounces each), rinsed and patted dry
- 1 tablespoon ancho chile powder
- 1¼ teaspoons sea salt, divided
- 2 jalapeño peppers, seeded and minced
- 4 garlic cloves, minced
- 8 strips applewood-smoked bacon
- 4 small sweet potatoes, unpeeled and cut into ½-inch dice
- 1 tablespoon olive oil

1. Preheat the oven to 450°F. Line a sheet pan with parchment paper.

2. Season the quail with the chile powder and 1 teaspoon of the sea salt inside and out. Divide the minced jalapeño and garlic among the birds and stuff each with 1 to 2 teaspoons.

3. Wrap each quail breast with the strip of bacon. Place the quail on the sheet pan.

4. Toss the sweet potatoes with the olive oil and remaining ¼ teaspoon sea salt, and spread them on the sheet pan around the quail.

5. Roast uncovered for 15 to 20 minutes, or until the quail are cooked through and the sweet potatoes are browned.

6. Allow to rest for 10 minutes before serving.

HONEY MUSTARD RABBIT AND RAINBOW CARROTS

The strong flavor of rabbit is often prepared with grainy mustard. When paired with honey and carrots, it's a sweet and delicious combination.

SERVES: 4   PREP TIME: 10 minutes   COOK TIME: 1 to 1¼ hours

3 tablespoons coconut oil

2 tablespoons honey or maple syrup

2 tablespoons whole-grain mustard

1 teaspoon curry powder

1 rabbit, cut into 8 pieces

1 pound rainbow carrots, with 2 inches of tops, halved lengthwise

sea salt

freshly ground pepper

1. Preheat the oven to 350°F. Line a sheet pan with parchment paper.

2. Whisk together 2 tablespoons of the coconut oil, honey or maple syrup, mustard, and curry powder. Spread it over the rabbit pieces. Spread the pieces out on the sheet pan.

3. Toss the carrots with the remaining 1 tablespoon of the coconut oil. Season with salt and pepper. Spread out on the sheet pan around the rabbit.

4. Roast uncovered for 1 to 1¼, hours until the rabbit reaches an internal temperature of 160°F. Brush the meat and carrots with the pan juices. Allow to rest for 10 minutes before serving.

MEXICAN-SPICED BRAISED SQUAB

The silky texture of the squab is offset beautifully by the pungent spices.

SERVES: 4   PREP TIME: 15 minutes   COOK TIME: 1 hour

1 teaspoon dried oregano

1 teaspoon chipotle chile powder

1 teaspoon ancho chile powder

1 teaspoon smoked paprika

2 teaspoons garlic puree

½ teaspoon sea salt

¼ cup olive oil

4 (14-ounce) squab, cleaned and patted dry

1 yellow onion, sliced in thick rings

1 green bell pepper, sliced in thick slices

2 small white potatoes, cut into large chunks

1 cup dry white wine

1. Preheat the oven to 500°F.

2. Combine the oregano, chipotle chile powder, ancho chile powder, paprika, garlic, and salt in a small bowl. Brush the squab with olive oil and then coat in the spice mixture.

3. Place the squab on the sheet pan and roast uncovered for 20 minutes. Remove the pan from the oven and reduce the heat to 325°F.

4. Add the onion, bell pepper, and potatoes to the pan and pour in the white wine. Cover the pan tightly with foil and return to the oven for 30 minutes. Baste with the wine, cover, and cook for another 15 minutes, or until cooked to an internal temperature of 165°F. Allow to rest for 10 minutes before serving.

TERIYAKI VENISON STEAKS WITH PARSNIPS AND ONIONS

During my adolescence, my best friend's family hunted and fished. This was their favorite recipe for venison steaks.

SERVES: 4   PREP TIME: 10 minutes   COOK TIME: 15 minutes

⅓ cup coconut aminos

1 tablespoon maple syrup or honey

1 tablespoon minced onion

4 garlic cloves, crushed

2 bay leaves

⅓ cup plus 3 tablespoons olive oil, divided

4 venison steaks, about 8 ounces each

4 parsnips, unpeeled cut into ½-inch-thick slices

1 yellow onion, thinly sliced

sea salt

freshly ground pepper

1. Mix the coconut aminos, maple syrup or honey, onion, garlic, bay leaves, and ⅓ cup of the olive oil in a large glass bowl. Add the venison steaks, cover, and marinate for at least 1 hour or up to 8 hours.

2. Preheat the broiler to high and place an oven rack about 8 inches from the element; the food should be about 5 inches from the element. Line a sheet pan with parchment paper.

3. Toss the parsnips and sliced onion with the remaining 3 tablespoons olive oil and season with salt and pepper. Spread them out on the sheet pan.

4. Remove the venison steaks from the marinade and place on the sheet pan, pushing the parsnips aside to make four spaces.

5. Broil for 10 minutes, brushing occasionally with the remaining marinade. Keep a close eye on the vegetables, turning occasionally, and remove when just beginning to brown.

6. Turn the venison and broil 5 minutes longer or to your desired level of doneness.

NIGHTSHADE-FREE

SPICED ANTELOPE CHUCK ROAST

Antelope has a more mild flavor than venison, leaving it open to a variety of seasoning options. Broken Arrow Ranch, which harvests antelope from a million acres in south Texas, recommends seasoning heavily with a Tex-Mex spice blend and then cooking at low heat until the meat is tender.

SERVES: 4   PREP TIME: 15 minutes, plus 8 hours for marinating   COOK TIME: 2 to 2½ hours

¼ cup plus 1 tablespoon olive oil

¼ cup red wine vinegar

1 yellow onion, diced

2 garlic cloves, peeled

1 jalapeño, minced

2 tablespoons tomato paste

1½ teaspoons dried oregano

2 tablespoons New Mexico chili powder

1 tablespoon ancho chile powder

1 tablespoon ground cumin

1 teaspoon sea salt

½ teaspoon freshly ground pepper

2 pounds antelope chuck roast

2 yellow onions, sliced into rings

4 plum tomatoes, quartered lengthwise

2 cups cubed butternut squash

1. Combine the olive oil, vinegar, onion, garlic, jalapeño, tomato paste, oregano, New Mexico chili powder, ancho chile powder, cumin, salt, and pepper in a blender and puree until mostly smooth. Spread the mixture on the chuck roast, cover, and refrigerate overnight.

2. Remove the meat from the refrigerator and allow to come to room temperature.

3. Preheat the oven to 450°F.

4. Set the roast on a sheet pan. Roast uncovered for 30 minutes. Reduce the oven temperature to 325°F. Toss the onions, tomatoes, and squash with the remaining tablespoon of oil and season with salt and pepper. Add to the sheet pan and cook for another 1 to 1½ hours, until the meat is very tender. Allow to rest for 20 minutes before slicing and serving.

COFFEE-RUBBED ELK STEAKS WITH CHARRED LEEKS

Coffee rubs are becoming increasingly popular for seasoning steaks. You can purchase them in specialty grocery stores or make your own for a fraction of the cost.

SERVES: 4 PREP TIME: 10 minutes COOK TIME: 15 minutes

¼ cup ground coffee

2 tablespoons coconut palm sugar

½ teaspoon smoked paprika

1 teaspoon ground coriander

1 teaspoon sea salt, plus more to taste

4 tablespoons olive oil, divided

4 elk steaks

2 bunches leeks, white and pale green parts only, sliced in half lengthwise

freshly ground pepper

1. Preheat the oven to 350°F.

2. Combine the coffee, palm sugar, paprika, coriander, and salt in a small bowl. Pat the elk steaks dry with a paper towel and coat with 2 tablespoons of the olive oil. Coat them in the spice rub and allow to rest at room temperature.

3. Place the leeks them on a large square of foil. Drizzle with the remaining 2 tablespoons olive oil and season with salt and pepper. Fold the foil into a loose package, place on the sheet pan and roast for about 45 to 55 minutes, until soft. Remove the pan from the oven and remove the leeks to a cutting board. Place an oven-safe baking rack on the sheet pan.

4. Preheat the broiler and place the oven rack about 8 inches from the heating element; the food should be about 5 inches from the element.

5. Place the leeks, cut-side up, and elk steaks on the baking rack. Broil for 5 minutes.

6. Remove the leeks to a serving platter. Flip the steaks and broil 5 minutes longer, until the meat reaches an internal temperature of 130° to 140°F. Allow the meat to rest for 10 minutes before serving with the leeks.

ROASTED WILD BOAR LEG WITH LEEKS AND CHERRY WINE SAUCE

My husband's parents lived in Germany for many years in a house bordering a forest filled with wild boar. At the time, I was pretty concerned (read: deathly afraid) about meeting one of them while hiking through the snow. But now, the idea of hunting boar sounds intriguing. Whether or not you hunt your dinner or pick it up from a butcher, this recipe will give the meat the attention it deserves.

SERVES: 4 to 6   PREP TIME: 15 minutes, plus 12 hours for brining   COOK TIME: 3 to 5 hours

4 cups full-bodied, dry red wine

1 cup dried cherries

1 bunch fresh thyme sprigs

2 tablespoons black peppercorns

1 tablespoon sea salt

¼ cup red wine vinegar

4- to 6-pound leg of wild boar

4 tablespoons olive oil, divided

4 leeks

2 tablespoons maple syrup

1. Bring the red wine, cherries, and thyme to a simmer in a small saucepan for 5 minutes. Remove the cherries and ½ cup of the wine to a glass jar and refrigerate.

2. Add the peppercorns and salt to the wine in the saucepan and allow the mixture to cool completely. Stir in the vinegar. Pour the mixture over the boar leg, turning to coat. You can do this in either a glass baking dish or a zip-top plastic bag. Allow to marinate overnight or up to 36 hours in the refrigerator.

3. Preheat the oven to 400°F. Remove the boar from the marinade and pat dry with paper towels. Rub with 2 tablespoons of the olive oil and place on a sheet pan. Roast uncovered for 15 minutes. Turn the oven temperature down to 250°F and roast for another 3 to 4 hours.

The internal temperature of the meat should reach between 160° and 170°F.

4. During the last hour of cooking, thoroughly rinse the leeks and halve them, cutting off the green parts. Toss with the remaining 2 tablespoons of olive oil and season with salt and pepper. Place them on the sheet pan around the meat and return to the oven.

5. When the meat has reached an internal temperature of at least 160°F, remove it from the oven and allow to rest for 20 minutes. Wrap the leeks in foil to retain heat.

6. While the meat rests, warm the reserved cherries and wine in a small saucepan and puree with an immersion blender. Season with salt and pepper, and stir in the maple syrup.

7. Slice the boar and place on a serving platter with the leeks. Pour the cherry sauce over the meat just before serving.

WILD PHEASANT WITH PARSNIPS AND BLACKBERRY GLAZE

When I lived in England, I tried to enjoy as many dishes as I could that I didn't see regularly on American restaurant menus. One Sunday after church, we visited this small pub near our house. I had seen wild pheasant roaming the fields and woods as we drove through the countryside, so it was pretty cool to be able to enjoy it at the restaurant.

SERVES: 4   PREP TIME: 10 minutes   COOK TIME: 45 minutes

2 wild pheasant, 2½ to 3 pounds each

3 tablespoons rendered bacon fat, divided

4 parsnips, peeled and cut into chunks

1 cup Blackberry Glaze (page 255)

sea salt

freshly ground black pepper

1. Preheat the oven to 425°F. Line a sheet pan with parchment paper.

2. Coat the pheasant liberally with 2 tablespoons of the bacon fat. Season with salt and pepper. Place them on the sheet pan. Toss the parsnips with the remaining 1 tablespoon bacon fat and spread on the sheet pan around the pheasant. Season with salt and pepper.

3. Roast uncovered for 45 minutes, or until the meat reaches an internal temperature of 165°F.

4. Serve with the Blackberry Glaze, gently warmed.

CALF LIVER AND ONIONS

Mature cow liver tends to have a stronger flavor profile than calf liver, but if you prefer it or that is all you can find, feel free to use it instead.

SERVES: 4   PREP TIME: 10 minutes   COOK TIME: 40 minutes

2 yellow onions, sliced in thin rings

8 ounces cremini mushrooms, sliced

4 tablespoons rendered bacon fat, melted, divided

1 pound calf liver

2 teaspoons fresh minced rosemary

sea salt

freshly ground pepper

1. Preheat the oven to 375°F. Line a sheet pan with parchment paper.

2. Spread the onions and mushrooms out on the sheet pan. Drizzle with all 3 tablespoons of the bacon fat. Season with salt and pepper. Roast uncovered for 20 minutes.

3. While the onions and mushrooms cook, rinse the calf liver under cool running water. Slice it in ½-inch-thick slices. Pat dry with a paper towel and coat in the remaining 1 tablespoon bacon fat. Season with rosemary, salt, and pepper. Place on top of the vegetables and cook until the liver reaches an internal temperature of 160°F, about 20 minutes.

NIGHTSHADE-FREE

BEEF KIDNEY STEW

Of all the times to purchase organic, grass-fed, pastured meat, this is it. Kidneys filter an animal's waste, so if an animal lived in confinement on a grain-based diet and a cocktail of drugs and hormones, the effects will show up in its kidneys. On the other hand, kidney from sustainably raised cows is low in toxins and a rich source of vitamin B12, riboflavin, iron, and selenium. This recipe is based on the classic French dish from legendary chef Jacques Pépin.

SERVES: 6   PREP TIME: 10 minutes   COOK TIME: 55 to 60 minutes

2 to 3 beef kidneys, cut into 1½-inch pieces

3 tablespoons rendered bacon fat

4 yellow onions, halved then cut into half circles

4 tablespoons minced garlic

1 pound new potatoes, halved

8 ounces cremini mushrooms, halved

2 teaspoons fresh thyme leaves

2 teaspoons dry mustard

1 cup dry white wine

sea salt

freshly ground pepper

1. Preheat the oven to 325°F.

2. Trim any fat and membranes from the kidneys. Spread the kidneys on the sheet pan along with the onions, garlic, potatoes, mushrooms, thyme, and mustard. Drizzle with rendered bacon fat and season generously with salt and pepper. Pour the white wine over the whole pan and then cover tightly with foil.

3. Cook for 45 to 50 minutes until tender. Remove the foil and allow to rest for a few minutes before serving.

BROILED LAMB KIDNEY

A long braise works well, but kidney can also be prepared quickly with a short time under the broiler. Just be careful not to overcook it. Enjoy over a simple salad of mixed greens with a squeeze of lemon juice.

SERVES: 2   PREP TIME: 10 minutes, plus 30 for marinating   COOK TIME: 8 minutes

- 2 lamb kidneys
- 2 tablespoons olive oil
- 1 teaspoon fresh thyme
- ¼ teaspoon dry mustard
- 1 teaspoon minced shallot
- ⅛ teaspoon sea salt
- 2 tablespoons macadamia oil
- 1 tablespoon gluten-free Worcestershire sauce
- 1 tablespoon hot sauce
- juice of 1 lemon
- freshly ground pepper

1. Slice the kidneys in half horizontally and remove the white inner parts, fat, and skin.

2. Combine the olive oil, thyme, mustard, shallots, and salt in a shallow dish. Marinate the cleaned kidneys in this mixture for 30 minutes at room temperature.

3. Preheat the broiler. Fit an oven-safe rack on the sheet pan and brush with oil.

4. Place the kidneys on the rack and broil for 5 minutes.

5. Whisk together the macadamia oil, Worcestershire sauce, hot sauce, and lemon juice. Baste both sides of the kidneys with this mixture, turn over, and broil for another 3 minutes until browned on the exterior. Season with salt and pepper.

GINGER CHICKEN HEARTS WITH BOK CHOY

Close your eyes and you'll imagine that chicken hearts are actually just the juiciest, most delicious dark meat you've ever tried. They're quick and easy, and loaded with nutrition.

SERVES: 2 to 4   PREP TIME: 10 minutes, plus 1 to 2 hours for marinating   COOK TIME: 15 to 20 minutes

1 tablespoon minced fresh ginger

1 tablespoon minced garlic

½ teaspoon red chile flakes

1 teaspoon sesame oil

2 tablespoons coconut aminos

½ teaspoon sea salt

1 ½ pounds chicken hearts

4 baby bok choy, roughly chopped

2 tablespoons toasted sesame seeds

¼ cup roughly chopped fresh cilantro

1. Combine the ginger, garlic, chile flakes, sesame oil, coconut aminos, and salt in a glass dish. Slice each of the chicken hearts into three pieces lengthwise and add them to the ginger mixture. Toss to coat thoroughly. Cover and refrigerate for 1 to 2 hours.

2. Preheat the oven to 425°F. Line a sheet pan with parchment paper. Spread the bok choy out on the sheet pan. Spread the marinated chicken hearts out over the bok choy.

3. Roast uncovered for 15 to 20 minutes, or until the chicken hearts are tender and cooked through.

4. To serve, top with the toasted sesame seeds and cilantro.

CUBAN-STYLE ROASTED CALF BRAIN TACOS

Brains require a bit more advance preparation than some other organ meats. They're typically fried and served as an appetizer in Cuba. Here is a Paleo-friendly adaptation.

SERVES: 2 PREP TIME: 20 minutes, plus 2 hours for soaking COOK TIME: 20 minutes

1 pair calf brains about 1 pound

3 tablespoons lime juice, divided

1 teaspoon sea salt, divided

2 tablespoons coconut oil

2 teaspoons ground cumin

1 teaspoon smoked paprika

8 savoy cabbage leaves

1 red onion, halved then sliced in thin circles

½ cup roughly chopped fresh cilantro

1. Soak the brains in cold water for 2 hours in the refrigerator. Remove as much of the filament and membranes as possible.

2. Bring a large pot of water to a simmer with the brains fully submerged. Stir in 1 tablespoon of the lime juice and ½ a teaspoon of the salt. Cook for 15 minutes, then set the brains on a cutting board to cool.

3. Preheat the oven to 425°F. Line a sheet pan with parchment paper.

4. Cut the brains into small chunks. Toss them with the coconut oil, remaining salt, cumin, and paprika. Spread them out on the sheet pan. Roast uncovered for 20 minutes, until browned.

5. To serve, place a spoonful of the calf brains into each cabbage leaf and top with red onion, cilantro, and a sprinkle of the remaining 2 tablespoons of lime juice.

SWEETBREADS AND MUSHROOMS

Mushrooms are a classic flavor pairing for sweetbreads. The organ meat is typically composed of the thymus, pancreas, or other glands.

SERVES: 2 to 4   PREP TIME: 20 minutes, plus 8 to 10 hours for soaking and pressing   COOK TIME: 15 minutes

1 pound sweetbreads	1 teaspoon fresh thyme
1 teaspoon lemon juice	½ cup dry white wine
2 tablespoons rendered bacon fat	salt
8 ounces cremini mushrooms, sliced ½ inch thick	freshly ground pepper

1. Soak the sweetbreads in cold water for 6 to 8 hours.

2. Bring a large pot of water to a simmer with the sweetbreads fully submerged. Stir in the lemon juice. Cook for 15 minutes, then plunge the sweetbreads into ice water. Remove as much of the veins, filament, and membranes as possible.

3. Place the sweetbreads in one layer on a clean towel. Top with another towel and place a heavy pot over it to press for at least 2 hours in the refrigerator.

4. Preheat the oven to 425°F.

5. Slice the sweetbreads into medallions about ½ to 1 inch thick. Place them in a shallow bowl and toss with the bacon fat, mushrooms, and thyme. Season with salt and pepper.

6. Spread the mixture out on the sheet pan.

7. Roast uncovered for 15 minutes. Pour in the white wine and cook for another 25 minutes, until most of the wine has evaporated, the exterior will be slightly browned and crisp and the interior, tender.

CHAPTER TEN

Desserts

RAW ENERGY BARS

While this recipe utilizes a sheet pan, it forgoes the oven altogether, which means less time to wait before you can slice into these yummy bars and enjoy them!

SERVES: 24   PREP TIME: 10 minutes   COOK TIME: none

1 cup shelled pistachios

1 cup pepitas (pumpkin seeds)

½ cup shelled hemp seeds

1 cup medjool dates, pitted

1 cup raisins

2 teaspoons maca powder (optional)

pinch of Himalayan pink sea salt

1 cup unsweetened shredded coconut

½ cup coconut oil

1. Combine all of the ingredients, except the coconut and coconut oil, in a food processor until crumbly and thoroughly integrated. Add the shredded coconut and pulse once or twice, just until combined. With the motor running, slowly drizzle in the coconut oil and continue blending until just combined.

2. Line a sheet pan with parchment paper. Spread the mixture evenly on the pan. Use another sheet of parchment to press the mixture into the pan.

3. Refrigerate for at least 30 minutes before slicing into bars. Store in the refrigerator for up to one week.

NIGHTSHADE-FREE ▪ VEGAN

CHOCOLATE ORANGE ENERGY BARS

Chocolate and orange are a match made in heaven in my book. When I was growing up, as gifts we received chocolate "oranges" with segments of delicious orange-scented chocolate wrapped in orange foil. These bars remind me of that candy, but they're so much healthier!

SERVES: 24   PREP TIME: 10 minutes   COOK TIME: none

1½ cups walnuts

1 cup almonds

1 cup Medjool dates, pitted

1 cup raisins

zest and juice of 1 orange

2 heaping tablespoons unsweetened cocoa powder

pinch of Himalayan pink sea salt

1. Combine all of the ingredients, except the orange juice, in a food processor until crumbly and thoroughly integrated. Add the orange juice and pulse until the mixture comes together.

2. Line a sheet pan with parchment paper. Spread the mixture evenly on the pan. Use another sheet of parchment to press the mixture into the pan.

3. Refrigerate for at least 30 minutes before slicing into bars. Store covered in the refrigerator for up to one week.

NIGHTSHADE-FREE • VEGAN

VANILLA COCONUT CONGO BARS

This dessert don't have the cake-like texture of some congo bars, but I think that makes them even better. Bonus: You don't even have to bake them! However, refrigeration is essential, especially if you make them in the middle of summer like I did the first time.

SERVES: 24   PREP TIME: 10 minutes   COOK TIME: none

3¼ cups chopped pecans, divided

¾ teaspoon Himalayan pink sea salt

3 tablespoons unsweetened cocoa powder

¾ cup medjool dates, pitted

1 cup coconut oil, in solid form

1 vanilla bean, split and scraped

½ cup maple syrup

2 cups unsweetened shredded coconut, divided

¼ cup cacao nibs

1. Line a sheet pan with parchment paper.

2. Combine 3 cups of the pecans, sea salt, cocoa powder, and dates in a food processor and pulse until relatively smooth. Press the mixture into the sheet pan; it will be about ½ inch thick. Store in the refrigerator while you continue with the filling.

3. In a large bowl, whisk together the coconut oil, vanilla bean seeds, and maple syrup until thoroughly combined. Stir in 1½ cups of the shredded coconut. Spread this mixture over the chocolate crust.

4. Sprinkle the remaining ¼ cup pecans, ½ cup coconut, and the cacao nibs over the coconut filling. Refrigerate for 1 hour before cutting and serving. Store loosely covered in the refrigerator for up to 3 days.

NIGHTSHADE-FREE • LOW-FODMAP • VEGAN

APPLE CRISP

This dessert is perfect when the weather finally starts to cool off in the evenings and the first apple harvest rolls in. Use whatever apples are available where you live. I enjoy Granny Smith, Braeburn, and Pink Lady apples for their balance of sweet and tart flavors.

SERVES: 6 to 8   PREP TIME: 15 minutes   COOK TIME: 30 to 45 minutes

8 apples, peeled, cored, and diced

4 tablespoons tapioca starch, divided

1 tablespoon ground cinnamon

½ teaspoon freshly grated nutmeg

1 cup blanched almond flour

¼ teaspoon sea salt

¼ cup coconut palm sugar

½ cup palm shortening

1. Preheat the oven to 350°F.

2. Combine the apples with 2 tablespoons of the tapioca starch and the cinnamon and nutmeg on a sheet pan.

3. In a food processor, combine the remaining 2 tablespoons tapioca starch, almond flour, salt, and palm sugar. Pulse once or twice, just to integrate all of the ingredients. Add the palm shortening by the spoonful to the food processor. Pulse a few times, or just until combined. Crumble the mixture over the apples.

4. Bake for 30 to 45 minutes, or until the apples are very soft and the top is browned.

NIGHTSHADE-FREE • VEGAN

BLUEBERRY CRISP

Every summer my mom received a postcard from Blueberry Hill Farm in rural Oregon letting us know that the blueberries were in season. We would pick all afternoon, my brothers and I racing to see who could fill up our buckets first. We came home with purple-hued fingers and a dozen pounds of fruit. My mom froze most of them and made delicious desserts like this one.

SERVES: 6 to 8   PREP TIME: 15 minutes   COOK TIME: 25 to 30 minutes

6 cups blueberries

4 tablespoons tapioca starch, divided

zest of 1 lemon

½ teaspoon freshly grated nutmeg

1 cup blanched almond flour

¼ teaspoon sea salt

¼ cup coconut palm sugar

½ cup palm shortening

1. Preheat the oven to 350°F.

2. Combine the blueberries with 2 tablespoons of the tapioca starch and the lemon zest on the sheet pan.

3. In a food processor, combine the remaining 2 tablespoons tapioca starch, almond flour, salt, and palm sugar. Pulse once or twice, just to integrate all of the ingredients. Add the palm shortening by the spoonful to the food processor. Pulse a few times, or just until combined. Crumble the mixture over the blueberries.

4. Bake for 25 to 30 minutes, or until the berries are soft and bubbling and the top is browned.

NIGHTSHADE-FREE ▪ LOW-FODMAP ▪ VEGAN

SHEET PAN PALEO

BLACKBERRY AND ROSEMARY CRISP

As a young newlywed, I received the book Tyler Florence's Real Kitchen *from my best friend Marcella. It was the only cookbook I had for a while, and I cooked nearly every recipe in it. I love the way he adds savory herbs to sweet dishes, particularly the combination of rosemary and blackberries here. This is my Paleo take on his dessert.*

SERVES: 6 to 8   PREP TIME: 5 minutes   COOK TIME: 30 minutes

2 pounds fresh blackberries, rinsed and dried

4 tablespoons tapioca starch, divided

1 cup blanched almond flour

¼ teaspoon sea salt

¼ cup coconut palm sugar

2 tablespoons fresh minced rosemary

½ cup palm shortening

1. Preheat the oven to 350°F.

2. Combine the blackberries with 2 tablespoons of the tapioca starch on the sheet pan.

3. In a food processor, combine the remaining tapioca starch, almond flour, salt, palm sugar, and rosemary. Pulse once or twice, just to integrate all of the ingredients. Add the palm shortening by the spoonful to the food processor. Pulse a few times, or just until combined. Crumble the mixture over the blackberries.

4. Bake for 30 minutes, or until the berries are very soft and the top is gently browned.

NIGHTSHADE-FREE ▪ VEGAN

BAKED NECTARINES WITH PISTACHIO FILLING

I love the tart juiciness of the nectarines offset by the salty, crunchy filling of pistachio mixture. Enjoy on its own or topped with a scoop of vanilla Paleo ice cream.

SERVES: 4   PREP TIME: 10 minutes   COOK TIME: 20 minutes

4 nectarines, halved and pitted

½ cup shelled pistachios

⅛ teaspoon Himalayan pink sea salt

2 tablespoons palm shortening

2 tablespoons coconut palm sugar

½ teaspoon vanilla extract

1. Preheat the oven to 350°F.

2. Arrange the nectarine halves on a sheet pan, cut-side up. If they fall over, slice a small portion of the bottom from each one or form a ring with aluminum foil to keep them upright.

3. Pulse the pistachios in a food processor until coarsely ground. You want some nut pieces remaining. Add the sea salt, palm shortening, palm sugar, and vanilla, and pulse until just combined. Divide the mixture among the nectarine halves.

4. Bake uncovered for 20 minutes until browned and bubbling. Allow to rest for 10 minutes before serving.

NIGHTSHADE-FREE ▪ VEGAN

ROASTED FIGS WITH ROSEMARY

This easy, healthy dessert is bursting with the flavors of summer. Roasting concentrates the natural sweetness of the figs, so I've added just a touch of coconut palm sugar. Serve with your favorite Paleo ice cream or enjoy chilled.

SERVES: 4   PREP TIME: 5 minutes   COOK TIME: 30 to 40 minutes

2 pounds fresh figs, quartered

1 sprig rosemary, needles minced

1 tablespoon coconut oil

2 tablespoons red wine

2 tablespoons maple syrup

1. Preheat the oven to 400°F. Line a sheet pan with parchment paper.

2. Combine all of the ingredients in a large bowl, tossing to coat thoroughly.

3. Spread the figs out on the sheet pan cut-side down and roast uncovered for 30 to 40 minutes, until the figs begin to caramelize but before the sugars burn on the pan. If you want juicier figs, cover with aluminum foil for the entire roasting time.

NIGHTSHADE-FREE ▪ VEGAN

BANANA COCONUT BARS

These make an awesome dessert or a healthy breakfast, especially if you're tired of the standard bacon and eggs. Anything made with bananas is an easy sell in my house—they're so popular with my kiddos, I've made it my goal to someday find myself with too many ripe bananas. It just doesn't happen.

MAKES: 24   PREP TIME: 15 minutes   COOK TIME: 35 to 40 minutes

4 eggs

3 ripe bananas

1 tablespoon vanilla extract

½ cup maple syrup

½ cup coconut milk

½ teaspoon sea salt

1 teaspoon ground cinnamon

¼ cup coconut flour

1 cup blanched almond flour

2 cups unsweetened shredded coconut, divided

1 cup finely chopped walnuts, divided

1. Preheat the oven to 350°F. Line a sheet pan with parchment paper, allowing it to come up the sides.

2. Combine the eggs, bananas, vanilla, maple syrup, and coconut milk in a blender and puree for 15 seconds, scraping down the sides once. Add the salt, cinnamon, coconut flour, and almond flour. Pulse a few times, scrape down the sides, then puree for 10 seconds.

3. Add 1 cup of the shredded coconut and ½ cup of the walnuts and pulse once or twice, just to combine.

4. Pour the mixture onto the sheet pan and top with the remaining coconut and walnuts. Bake for 35 to 40 minutes, or until the mixture is set but not overly browned. Allow to cool for at least 15 minutes before slicing.

NIGHTSHADE-FREE ▪ LOW-FODMAP

RASPBERRY ALMOND BARS

These bars are perfect to add to school lunches. Unlike most kid treats, they're not loaded with artificial colors, flavors, and high-fructose corn syrup.

MAKES: 24   PREP TIME: 15 minutes   COOK TIME: 35 to 40 minutes

4 eggs

1 tablespoon vanilla extract

½ cup maple syrup, divided

⅔ cup coconut milk

½ teaspoon sea salt

¼ cup coconut flour

1½ cups blanched almond flour

1½ cups unsweetened shredded coconut, divided

2 cups raspberries

1 cup sliced almonds

1. Preheat the oven to 350°F. Line a sheet pan with parchment paper, allowing it to come up the sides.

2. Combine the eggs, vanilla, ⅓ cup of the maple syrup, and coconut milk in a blender and puree for 15 seconds, scraping down the sides once. Add the salt, coconut flour, and almond flour. Pulse a few times, scrape down the sides, and then puree for 10 seconds.

3. Add 1 cup of the shredded coconut and pulse once or twice, just to combine.

4. Pour the mixture onto the sheet pan. Bake for 25 minutes.

5. Meanwhile, puree the raspberries and press through a fine mesh sieve. Whisk together with the remaining maple syrup.

6. Remove the sheet pan from the oven and drizzle with the raspberry puree. Sprinkle the almonds and remaining coconut over the top. Return to the oven to cook for another 15 minutes.

7. Allow to cool for at least 15 minutes before slicing.

NIGHTSHADE-FREE • LOW-FODMAP

COCONUT LIME PIE BARS

I love the tropical flavors in this cool and creamy dessert. Make sure to find unsweetened shredded coconut and invest the extra few minutes to toast it. It really adds a lovely depth of flavor.

MAKES: 24   PREP TIME: 15 minutes   COOK TIME: 10 to 12 minutes

1 ½ cups unsweetened coconut flakes, divided

2 cups blanched almonds

½ teaspoon Himalayan pink sea salt

¾ cup medjool dates

2 (15-ounce) cans coconut cream

zest and juice of 6 limes

¼ cup maple syrup

1. Preheat the broiler. Spread the coconut flakes on a sheet pan and toast for 1 to 2 minutes until lightly golden. Be careful not to burn them. Remove the pan from the oven and turn the oven temperature to 350°F.

2. Combine the almonds, sea salt, and dates in a food processor and process until coarsely ground. Add 1 cup of the toasted coconut flakes and pulse until just integrated.

3. Line the sheet pan with parchment paper and press the almond and coconut mixture into it with your hands. Bake uncovered for about 10 to 12 minutes, or until lightly toasted. Allow to cool completely.

4. Combine the coconut cream, lime zest and juice, and maple syrup in a large bowl and beat until light and fluffy. Spread the cream out over the crust and top with the remaining toasted coconut. Place the pan into the freezer for about an hour to set, then slice into bars and serve. Store covered in the refrigerator for up to 3 days.

NIGHTSHADE-FREE ▪ VEGAN

DENSE FUDGY BROWNIES

No, cavemen probably didn't sit around a fire chomping on brownies, but I'm convinced they would have if they had tried these. They are delicious as is or topped with whipped coconut cream with a hint of vanilla.

MAKES: 24   PREP TIME: 10 minutes   COOK TIME: 25 to 30 minutes

2/3 cup maple syrup

¼ cup palm shortening

3 eggs

1 tablespoon vanilla extract

2 cups almond butter

1 teaspoon baking soda

½ teaspoon sea salt

⅔ cup good-quality cocoa powder

1. Preheat the oven to 325°F. Line a sheet pan with parchment paper, making sure it goes up the sides of the pan.

2. Beat the maple syrup and palm shortening until thoroughly emulsified. Add the eggs and vanilla and beat until smooth. Beat in the almond butter.

3. In a small bowl, sift together the baking soda, sea salt, and cocoa powder. Add it to the wet ingredients, beating until just combined.

4. Pour the mixture into the sheet pan, smoothing it out until it reaches the sides. Bake for 25 to 30 minutes. Allow to cool for 15 minutes before slicing.

NIGHTSHADE-FREE ▪ LOW-FODMAP

PORT-SOAKED CHERRY BROWNIES

I met Iron Chef *judge and cookbook author Candace Kumai at an event in Hollywood where she gave me a copy of her book* Cook Yourself Sexy. *I absolutely love it and have had my eyes on her port-soaked cherry brownies since then, but I wanted to figure out how to make them without grain flours and butter. Here's my Paleo-friendly version.*

MAKES: 24   PREP TIME: 10 minutes, plus overnight to macerate   COOK TIME: 25 to 30 minutes

2 cups fresh pitted cherries

1 cup dried cherries

1 cup port

1 cup palm shortening

8 ounces dark chocolate, at least 80 percent cocoa

6 eggs

¾ cup coconut palm sugar

1 tablespoon vanilla extract

2 cups blanched almond flour

½ cup unsweetened cocoa powder

1 teaspoon baking powder

1½ teaspoons sea salt

1. Combine the fresh and dried cherries with the port and allow to macerate overnight in the refrigerator. Strain the fruit and reserve the port for another use (such as a port reduction).

2. Preheat the oven to 350°F. Line a sheet pan with parchment paper so that it comes up the sides.

3. Melt the palm shortening and dark chocolate over very low heat in a heavy skillet. Allow to cool.

4. In a large bowl, beat the eggs, palm sugar, and vanilla. In a medium bowl, sift together the almond flour, cocoa powder, baking powder, and salt. Stir in the melted chocolate, then fold in the cherries.

5. Spread the mixture out in the sheet pan smoothing until it reaches the edges. Bake uncovered for 25 to 30 minutes until set.

CLASSIC COFFEE CAKE

I grew up with the amazing Entenmann's pastries that were so full of sugar, just one slice sent me and my brothers into orbit. This is my grain-free take on their classic crumb cake. It contains far less sugar and no preservatives.

SERVES: 24   PREP TIME: 10 minutes   COOK TIME: 30 to 35 minutes

1 cup coconut palm sugar

½ cup palm shortening

5 eggs

1 tablespoon vanilla extract

4 cups blanched almond flour

1 teaspoon ground cinnamon

½ teaspoon sea salt

For the Topping:

¼ cup palm shortening

¼ cup coconut palm sugar

2 tablespoon almond flour

1 tablespoon ground cinnamon

¼ teaspoon sea salt

1. Preheat the oven to 350°F. Line a sheet pan with parchment paper, making sure it goes up the sides of the pan.

2. Beat the palm sugar and shortening until thoroughly emulsified. Add the eggs and vanilla and beat until smooth.

3. In a large bowl, sift together the almond flour, cinnamon, and sea salt. Add it to the wet ingredients, beating until just combined.

4. Pour the mixture into the sheet pan, smoothing it out until it reaches the sides.

5. To make the topping, combine all of the ingredients in a small food processor, or simply mash together with a fork. Crumble the mixture over the cake batter.

6. Bake for 30 to 35 minutes or until the edges are browned and the center is set. Allow to cool for 15 minutes before slicing.

NIGHTSHADE-FREE ▪ LOW-FODMAP

CHOCOLATE-COVERED FROZEN BANANA CHIPS

The sheet pan functions like an anti-griddle in this simple frozen dessert. The only thing it really requires is patience—these are so delicious you'll want to gobble them up before they're done!

MAKES: 36 chips   PREP TIME: 10 minutes, plus 30 minutes for freezing
COOK TIME: none

2 ripe bananas

½ cup coconut oil

¼ cup unsweetened cocoa powder

1 tablespoon maple syrup

fine sea salt

1. Line a sheet pan with parchment paper.

2. Slice the bananas in ⅛-inch-thick slices and place them in a single layer on the sheet pan. Place it in the freezer for about 30 minutes, until the bananas are firm but not completely frozen.

3. Meanwhile, whisk together the coconut oil, cocoa powder, maple syrup, and a pinch of fine sea salt in a shallow bowl.

4. Dip the frozen banana slices one at a time in the coconut-cocoa mixture and place them back on the sheet pan. Return the pan to the freezer for 10 minutes before enjoying.

NIGHTSHADE-FREE · LOW-FODMAP · VEGAN

PALEO THIN MINTS

I was undone when I tasted the filling for these cookies the first time and thought it couldn't get any better. And then I decided to dip them in a chocolate shell coating. This is my new favorite dessert recipe.

MAKES: 2 dozen cookies   PREP TIME: 10 minutes, plus 25 minutes for freezing   COOK TIME: none

1 cup medjool dates, pitted

1 cup walnuts

¼ cup plus 3 tablespoons cocoa powder, divided

¼ teaspoon peppermint oil

1 tablespoon cacao nibs

½ cup coconut oil

1 tablespoon maple syrup

sea salt

1. Combine the dates and walnuts in a food processor and process until fairly smooth. Add 3 tablespoons of the cocoa powder and a pinch of sea salt and pulse until thoroughly integrated. Sprinkle in the peppermint oil and pulse several more times. Finally, add the cacao nibs and pulse once or twice more, just until integrated.

2. Line a sheet pan with parchment paper. Form the dough into small, flat cookie shapes and place them on the pan. Place the pan in the freezer for 20 minutes. You do not want to freeze the cookies, just thoroughly chill them. If you want to make the filling ahead of time, simply store the cookies in the refrigerator until ready to coat with the chocolate.

3. Meanwhile, whisk together the remaining ¼ cup cocoa powder, coconut oil, maple syrup, and another tiny pinch of sea salt in a shallow bowl.

4. One at a time, dunk the cookies into the chocolate oil, shaking off any excess, and return to the sheet pan.

5. Place in the freezer for 5 minutes just to firm up again. If for some reason you don't eat them all in one sitting, store the cookies in the refrigerator for up to 3 days.

NIGHTSHADE-FREE ▪ LOW-FODMAP ▪ VEGAN

DUTCH BABIES

My father traveled for business occasionally when I was growing up, and whenever he did my mom would make us Dutch babies for dinner. Yes, for dinner. Whatever meal you enjoy these for, you're in for a treat!

SERVES: 4   PREP TIME: 5 minutes   COOK TIME: 25 to 28 minutes

¼ cup coconut oil

1 dozen eggs

1 cup full-fat coconut milk

1 tablespoon vanilla extract

4 tablespoons maple syrup, divided

½ cup tapioca starch

¼ cup coconut flour

½ teaspoon salt

fresh berries, for serving

1. Preheat oven to 400°F.

2. Coat the bottom and sides of a sheet pan with coconut oil and place in the oven while it preheats.

3. Place the eggs, coconut milk, vanilla, and 2 tablespoons of the maple syrup in the blender and blend until smooth. Add the tapioca starch, coconut flour, and salt and blend until smooth, scraping down the sides once or twice.

4. Pour the batter into the preheated pan and cook for 25 to 28 minutes, or until golden and puffy.

5. Drizzle the remaining 2 tablespoons of maple syrup over the Dutch babies when they come out of the oven and serve with fresh berries.

NIGHTSHADE-FREE ▪ LOW-FODMAP

BROILED SALTED VANILLA GRAPEFRUIT

I have always had a sour tooth and began enjoying grapefruit as a child. At the time, I smothered it in honey and ate it with a spoon. Here is a grownup version that makes for a decadent dessert. Don't skip the salt—it virtually erases any hint of bitterness in the fruit and will convert even the most ardent grapefruit skeptic.

SERVES: 8   PREP TIME: 10 minutes   COOK TIME: 7 minutes

4 ruby red grapefruit, halved

½ teaspoon Himalayan pink sea salt

2 teaspoons vanilla extract

4 tablespoons coconut palm sugar

1. Preheat the broiler. Place the oven rack on the top, about 5 inches from the element.

2. Use a paring knife to cut around the inside of each grapefruit half and between the segments; this makes it easier to remove after broiling. Place the grapefruit on a sheet pan.

3. Sprinkle each grapefruit half with a tiny pinch of sea salt then drizzle with ¼ teaspoon of the vanilla. Top each with ½ tablespoon of the coconut palm sugar.

4. Place the grapefruit under the broiler for 7 minutes, or until browned and bubbling. Allow to rest for a few minutes before serving.

NIGHTSHADE-FREE · VEGAN

BLACKBERRY BLUEBERRY HAND PIES

Every summer, my family and I picked blackberries, which grow abundantly throughout the Northwest, where I grew up. I recently introduced my younger son to the tradition so we could make this awesome blackberry and blueberry pie filling. It was well worth all the berry stains and thorns! It's delicious with a Paleo vanilla ice cream or whipped coconut cream.

SERVES: 6 to 8   PREP TIME: 15 minutes   COOK TIME: 40 to 45 minutes

4 cups fresh blackberries

2 cups fresh blueberries

zest of 1 lemon

1¼ teaspoons sea salt, divided

2 tablespoons coconut palm sugar

5 tablespoons tapioca flour, divided

4 cups blanched almond flour

5 tablespoons ice water

¼ cup palm shortening

1 large egg

1. Combine the berries, lemon zest, ¼ teaspoon of the sea salt, palm sugar, and 3 tablespoons of the tapioca flour in a large bowl. Allow to rest for a few minutes while you make the pastry dough.

2. Combine the almond flour, remaining 2 tablespoons of the tapioca flour, and remaining 1 teaspoon sea salt in a food processor and pulse once or twice. Add the ice water, palm shortening, and egg, and blend until thoroughly combined. Divide the mixture into 6 to 8 small balls and place in the refrigerator.

3. Preheat the oven to 325°F. Line a sheet pan with parchment paper.

4. Remove the pastry from the refrigerator and roll a ball of dough between two sheets of parchment until it is a thin circle. Remove the top square of parchment.

5. Place some of the berry filling on the center of the pastry circle, slightly to one side. Pick up the parchment paper to fold the other side over and press the seam together. Carefully transfer the pie to the sheet pan. Make a thin slit in the top of the pie for steam to escape. Repeat with the remaining pastry dough.

6. Bake uncovered for 40 to 45 minutes.

NIGHTSHADE-FREE ▪ VEGAN

BANANAS FOSTER

To the purists out there, I'm sorry. This isn't a true bananas foster. There are no flames and I've forgone the copious amounts of sugar. But the flavors are absolutely exquisite.

SERVES: 4   PREP TIME: 5 minutes   COOK TIME: 15 minutes

¼ cup coconut palm sugar

¼ teaspoon ground allspice

½ teaspoon freshly grated nutmeg

zest of 1 orange

2 tablespoons coconut oil

¼ cup dark rum

4 ripe bananas, sliced in half lengthwise

Paleo vanilla ice cream or crepes, for serving

1. Preheat the oven to 400°F. Place the oven rack about five inches from the top. Line a sheet pan with parchment paper.

2. Combine the palm sugar, allspice, nutmeg, orange zest, coconut oil, and rum in a shallow dish and stir to dissolve the sugar.

3. Soak the bananas in the liquid, turning to coat thoroughly. Place them on the sheet pan, cut-side down. Bake for 10 minutes. Remove the pan from the oven, turn the bananas over, and baste with the pan sauces. Switch the oven to broil. Broil the bananas for 3 to 4 minutes. Serve with a Paleo vanilla ice cream or crepes.

NIGHTSHADE-FREE · LOW-FODMAP · VEGAN

CHAPTER ELEVEN

Sauces

ROASTED TOMATO MARINARA SAUCE

There are numerous reasons to avoid canned foods, and the amazing flavor you'll find in this fresh tomato sauce is the most compelling. It is complex and sweet without even a pinch of added sugar. If you're making it in late summer when tomatoes are in abundance, definitely make an extra pan or two to freeze for later.

MAKES: 4 cups   PREP TIME: 5 minutes   COOK TIME: 1 hour

3 pounds fresh tomatoes, larger ones halved

2 to 3 shallots, quartered

4 to 6 garlic cloves

1 tablespoon fresh thyme leaves

1 tablespoon fresh oregano leaves

2 tablespoons olive oil

sea salt

freshly ground pepper

1. Preheat the oven to 350°F. Line a sheet pan with parchment paper.

2. Spread the tomatoes, shallots, garlic, thyme, and oregano out on the sheet pan. Drizzle the olive oil over the top and season with salt and pepper. Toss gently to coat. Roast uncovered for about 1 hour, or until the tomatoes are soft and barely browned.

3. Allow the tomatoes to cool before placing them into a blender. Puree until smooth, then press through a fine mesh sieve to remove the skins and seeds. If you prefer a chunky sauce, puree only half of the mixture and then stir in the remaining half.

VEGAN

BARBECUE SAUCE

I could eat virtually anything if it were coated in enough barbecue sauce. Problem is, most commercially prepared barbecue sauces are loaded with questionable ingredients, such as high-fructose corn syrup, MSG, and artificial flavors. Try this one and you'll never go back to those store-bought varieties! Enjoy it with Cowboy Meatballs and Onions (page 154).

MAKES: 2 to 3 cups   PREP TIME: 5 minutes   COOK TIME: 20 minutes

2 tablespoons coconut oil

1 yellow onion, minced

2 garlic cloves, minced

1 (15-ounce) can tomato sauce

1 tablespoon Dijon mustard

1 tablespoon chipotle chile powder

1 teaspoon ground cumin

2 teaspoons smoked paprika

¼ cup sherry vinegar or red wine vinegar

2 tablespoons coconut palm sugar

sea salt

freshly ground pepper

1. Warm the coconut oil over medium heat in a small saucepan. Add the onions and garlic and cook until soft, about 10 minutes.

2. Add the remaining ingredients and season with salt and pepper. Allow to simmer over low heat for 10 minutes.

VEGAN

QUICK PALEO MOLE

Traditional mole uses corn tortillas or bread to thicken the sauce. This Paleo-friendly version thickens naturally as it loses moisture during the long roasting time when prepared with Roasted Chicken Mole with Baked Sweet Potatoes (page 104).

MAKES: 2½ to 3 cups   PREP TIME: 10 minutes   COOK TIME: 40 minutes

4 dried poblano chile peppers

4 dried ancho chile peppers

2 cups chicken broth, heated

¼ cup raisins

½ cup sesame seeds

4 tablespoons coconut oil, divided

1 yellow onion, minced

2 garlic cloves, minced

½ teaspoon ground cloves

1 teaspoon ground cinnamon

1 teaspoon ground coriander

1 teaspoon ground anise seed or fennel seed

1 teaspoon freshly ground pepper

¼ cup blanched almonds

¼ cup pepitas (pumpkin seeds)

3 ounces very dark chocolate, grated

sea salt

1. Remove the seeds and stems from the chile peppers. Toast them in a hot skillet for about 30 seconds on each side, flattening with the back of a wooden spoon. Roughly chop them, then place in a blender along with the heated chicken broth and raisins to soften.

2. Toast the sesame seeds in a dry skillet over medium heat until fragrant and golden. Add to the blender.

3. Heat 2 tablespoons of the coconut oil in the same skillet and cook the onions until soft, about 10 minutes. Add the garlic, cloves, cinnamon, coriander, anise or fennel, and pepper, and continue cooking for another 2 minutes. Transfer to the blender.

4. Heat the remaining 2 tablespoons coconut oil in the skillet and cook the almonds and pepitas for 5 minutes. Transfer to the blender.

5. Puree the ingredients in the blender until smooth. Season with salt. Transfer the sauce to a medium saucepan over medium heat and simmer uncovered for 20 minutes, then stir in the dark chocolate. Allow to cool before storing in a covered container in the refrigerator.

CABERNET BARBECUE SAUCE

This sauce combines the richness of a wine reduction with an every-day barbecue sauce to brilliant effect. It's amazing spread over grilled meat or the Rosemary, Onion, and Potato Pie (page 61).

MAKES: 1 cup   PREP TIME: 5 minutes   COOK TIME: 15 to 20 minutes

1 tablespoon olive oil

2 tablespoons minced onion

2 garlic cloves, minced

1 sprig fresh thyme

1 cup Cabernet

½ cup tomato sauce

1 teaspoon Dijon mustard

½ teaspoon smoked paprika

1 teaspoon coconut palm sugar

sea salt

freshly ground pepper

1. Warm the olive oil in a small saucepan over medium-low heat. Add the onion and garlic and cook for about 10 minutes, until softened. Add the thyme and Cabernet, and simmer for 10 to 15 minutes, until reduced by half. Discard the thyme sprig.

2. Stir in the remaining ingredients and bring to a gentle simmer for a few minutes. Season with salt and pepper.

SALSA VERDE

I love the tang of tomatillos and roasted garlic and onion in this awesome salsa. Feel free to adjust the amount of serrano chile in accordance with your heat preferences.

MAKES: 4 to 6 cups   PREP TIME: 5 minutes   COOK TIME: 20 to 30 minutes

4 cups tomatillos, husked and rinsed

1 red onion, thinly sliced

4 garlic cloves

1 serrano chile, quartered lengthwise

2 tablespoons olive oil

sea salt

juice of 1 lime

½ cup roughly chopped fresh cilantro

1. Preheat the oven to 400°F. Line a sheet pan with parchment paper.

2. Spread the tomatillos, onion, garlic, and serrano chile out on the sheet pan. Toss with the olive oil and season with salt. Roast uncovered for 20 to 30 minutes, or until the tomatillos are tender but before the onions brown.

3. Allow the mixture to cool, and then transfer to a blender along with the lime juice and cilantro. Puree until mostly smooth.

VEGAN

PICO DE GALLO

This simple raw salsa can easily be purchased from a local grocery store, but tomatoes lose so much flavor when they're refrigerated, and many store-bought versions contain preservatives.

MAKES: 4 to 5 cups   PREP TIME: 10 minutes   COOK TIME: none

4 cups diced ripe tomatoes

2 garlic cloves, minced

1 shallot, minced

1 jalapeño pepper, minced

zest and juice of 2 limes

½ cup minced fresh cilantro

sea salt

freshly ground pepper

1. Combine all of the ingredients in a small bowl. Season with salt and pepper.

2. Cover and leave at room temperature until ready to serve to allow the flavors to come together.

PALEO MAYONNAISE

Commercially prepared mayonnaise is loaded with industrial oils such as safflower, soybean, and canola. All are loaded with inflammatory omega-6 fats and have been processed with chemical solvents. Fortunately, once you make your own mayo at home, you'll realize just how easy it is to create a healthy version.

MAKES: ½ cup   PREP TIME: 5 minutes   COOK TIME: none

1 egg yolk

1 teaspoon white wine vinegar

pinch of sea salt

½ cup macadamia nut oil

1. Whisk the egg yolk, vinegar, and sea salt in a small bowl for about 30 seconds.

2. Slowly drizzle in the macadamia nut oil a drop or two at a time, whisking constantly. The mixture will thicken as you add the oil. Keep whisking until it is all incorporated.

NIGHTSHADE-FREE • LOW-FODMAP

BACON MAYO

This thick, creamy mayonnaise is plain and simple: awesome sauce. Surprisingly, the bacon flavor does not overwhelm the sauce. If you want a mayo without bacon specks, make sure to strain the fat through a metal sieve lined with a layer of cheesecloth. Use the mayo on Bison Burgers (page 178) or as a base for other sauces. Thanks to the saturated fat in the bacon, this sauce becomes solid when stored in the refrigerator, so plan to make it just before you want to use it.

MAKES: ½ cup   PREP TIME: 5 minutes   COOK TIME: none

1 egg yolk

½ teaspoon lemon juice

pinch of sea salt

½ cup rendered bacon fat, melted but not hot

1. Whisk the egg yolk, lemon juice, and sea salt in a small bowl for about 30 seconds.

2. Slowly drizzle in the bacon fat a drop or two at a time, whisking constantly. The mixture will thicken as you add the fat. Keep whisking until it is all incorporated.

NIGHTSHADE-FREE • LOW-FODMAP

CILANTRO CREMA

This sauce is epic over Fish Tacos with Sweet Potatoes (page 75) and Spicy Asian Crab Cakes (page 88). It's also a delicious dip for sweet potato fries or drizzled over your favorite salad.

MAKES: 1 cup   PREP TIME: 5 minutes   COOK TIME: none

½ cup Paleo Mayonnaise (page 251)

juice of 3 limes

1 cup roughly chopped fresh cilantro

1. Combine the mayonnaise, lime juice, and cilantro in a blender and puree until smooth.

2. Will keep in the refrigerator for 2 days.

SWEET THAI CHILI SAUCE

This awesome chili sauce has just the right amount of sweet, sour, and salty flavors. Use it as a dipping sauce or to coat the Spicy Chili-Glazed Salmon with Mashed Plantains and Garlic (page 67).

MAKES: ½ cup   PREP TIME: 5 minutes   COOK TIME: 5 minutes

¼ cup rice wine vinegar

2 tablespoons fish sauce

2 tablespoons maple syrup

zest and juice of 1 lime

1 teaspoon minced garlic

1 teaspoon red chile flakes

1 teaspoon tapioca starch dissolved in 1 tablespoon water

1. Combine all of the ingredients, except the tapioca slurry, in a small saucepan and bring to a simmer for 5 minutes.

2. Stir in the tapioca slurry and cook until just thickened. Cool completely and store in a glass jar.

BLACKBERRY GLAZE

This sauce is delicious with Wild Pheasant with Parsnips (page 214) and roasted duck legs.

MAKES: 1 cup   PREP TIME: 5 minutes   COOK TIME: 20 minutes

2 cups fresh blackberries

1 tablespoon coconut palm sugar

pinch of sea salt

1 teaspoon minced fresh rosemary

1 teaspoon tapioca pearls

1. Combine the blackberries, palm sugar, sea salt, and rosemary in a small saucepan and bring to a gentle simmer. Cook for about 15 minutes, until pulpy and completely broken down.

2. Strain the mixture through a fine mesh sieve to remove the seeds and herbs and return to the stove.

3. Stir in the tapioca pearls and cook over low heat for about 5 minutes, until thickened.

PORT REDUCTION

Reducing wine and port concentrates their natural sweetness and imparts a tangy, slightly musty flavor. Serve this with the Pepper-Brined Pork Chops with Radicchio (page 136). Be very careful to cook it low and slow so you don't scorch the port.

MAKES: ½ cup   PREP TIME: 5 minutes   COOK TIME: 30 minutes

2 tablespoons olive oil

1 shallot, minced

1 garlic clove, minced

1 sprig thyme

½ cup chicken broth

½ cup red wine

1 cup port

1. Warm the olive oil over medium-low heat in a small saucepan. Add the shallot, garlic, and thyme and cook for about 10 minutes, until soft.

2. Add the chicken broth and red wine, and simmer until reduced to a few tablespoons. This will take at least 10 minutes.

3. Pour in the port and slowly reduce by about half. Discard the thyme. Allow to cool completely before storing in a covered container in the refrigerator.

NIGHTSHADE-FREE

PALEO BÉARNAISE SAUCE

Traditional béarnaise sauce is made with butter, but a similar flavor can be achieved with a pinch of salt and macadamia nut oil. Like most Hollandaise sauces, this one should be made just before serving. It is delicious with Whole Baked Trout with Lemon, Fennel, and Rainbow Carrots (page 70).

MAKES: ½ cup   PREP TIME: 5 minutes   COOK TIME: 15 minutes

1 bunch tarragon

1 shallot, minced

¼ cup white wine vinegar

¼ cup dry white wine

¼ teaspoon sea salt

3 egg yolks

6 tablespoons macadamia nut oil

1. Combine all but 1 sprig of the tarragon in a small saucepan with the shallots, vinegar, wine, and salt. Simmer for 10 minutes over low heat until reduced to just a few tablespoons.

2. Discard the tarragon sprigs and allow the mixture to cool for a minute or two. Add the egg yolk and whisk until the mixture begins to thicken.

3. Slowly drizzle in the macadamia nut oil a drop at a time until all of it is incorporated.

4. Mince the remaining sprig of tarragon and stir it into the sauce.

NIGHTSHADE-FREE

CLASSIC FRENCH RED WINE DEMI-GLACE

Many modern demi-glace recipes are thickened with flour and butter, decidedly not Paleo and frankly not very authentic either. Fortunately, the classic French sauce is made with, drumroll please, veal bone stock. Um, yes please! So, if you have the time to keep an eye on the stove, give this recipe a try. You can even store it in the freezer to keep it available for future use. Enjoy with Beef Rib Roast with New Potatoes (page 174).

MAKES: 2 cups   PREP TIME: 10 minutes   COOK TIME: 8 to 10 hours

1 pound veal bones

1 teaspoon red wine vinegar

4 cups cold water

1 cup diced yellow onion

½ cup diced carrots

½ cup celery

2 cups red wine

1. Preheat the oven to 400°F. Spread the veal bones out on a sheet pan and roast uncovered until browned, about 20 minutes.

2. Place the bones into a stock pot with the vinegar, cold water, onion, carrots, and celery. Cover and cook over medium heat for 4 to 6 hours. Strain the mixture and discard the vegetables and bones.

3. Return the liquid to the pan and cook uncovered until reduced by half.

4. Add the red wine and reduce by half again. The reduction process will take several hours. Be patient and enjoy the beautiful aromas filling your house.

Resources

Broken Arrow Ranch
www.brokenarrowranch.com
Pastured and wild game meats

Primal Kitchen
http://primalkitchen.com
Paleo-friendly mayonnaise

Not Ketchup
www.notketchup.com
Paleo-friendly sauces

D'Artagnan
www.dartagnan.com
Organic and free-range meats
and demi-glace

Wild Idea Buffalo
www.wildideabuffalo.com
Free-range bison meat

Barcelona's Gourmet Foods
http://www.barcelonasauces.com
Sauces such as Paleo-friendly
mole

FOR MORE INFORMATION ON
PALEO EATING:

Mark's Daily Apple
www.marksdailyapple.com
Science-based posts about
primal food and lifestyle, along
with testimonials

Chris Kresser
https://chriskresser.com
Medical perspective on the Paleo
diet.

*Perfect Health Diet: Regain
Health and Lose Weight by
Eating the Way You Were Meant
to Eat*, by Paul Jaminet, PhD and
Shou-Ching Jaminet, PhD

*Your Personal Paleo Code: The
3-Step Plan to Lose Weight,
Reverse Disease, and Stay Fit
and Healthy for Life*, by Chris
Kresser

Conversions

Temperature Conversions

Fahrenheit (°F)	Celsius (°C)
325°F	165°C
350°F	175°C
375°F	190°C
400°F	200°C
425°F	220°C
450°F	230°C

Volume Conversions

U.S.	U.S. equivalent	Metric
1 tablespoon (3 teaspoons)	½ fluid ounce	15 milliliters
¼ cup	2 fluid ounces	60 milliliters
⅓ cup	3 fluid ounces	90 milliliters
½ cup	4 fluid ounces	120 milliliters
⅔ cup	5 fluid ounces	150 milliliters
¾ cup	6 fluid ounces	180 milliliters
1 cup	8 fluid ounces	240 milliliters
2 cups	16 fluid ounces	480 milliliters

Weight Conversions

U.S.	Metric
½ ounce	15 grams
1 ounce	30 grams
2 ounces	60 grams
¼ pound	115 grams
⅓ pound	150 grams
½ pound	225 grams
¾ pound	350 grams
1 pound	450 grams

SHEET PAN **PALEO**

About the Author

Pamela Ellgen is a food blogger and cookbook author of *Soup & Comfort: A Cookbook of Homemade Soups to Warm the Soul* and *Modern Family Table: Savoring Fresh, Whole Foods with the People You Love*. She also writes on fitness and nutrition, and her work has appeared on LIVESTRONG, Spinning.com, and the Huffington Post. When she's not in the kitchen, Pamela enjoys surfing, practicing yoga, and playing with her kids. She lives in California with her husband and two children.